Dementia and Social Inclusion

of related interest

Healing Arts Therapies and Person-centred Dementia Care
Edited by Anthea Innes and Karen Hatfield
Bradford Dementia Group Good Practice Guides
ISBN 978 1 84310 038 6

Training and Development for Dementia Care Workers
Anthea Innes
Bradford Dementia Group Good Practice Guides
ISBN 978 1 85302 761 1

Understanding Dementia
The Man with the Worried Eyes
Richard Cheston and Michael Bender
ISBN 978 1 85302 479 5

Hearing the Voice of People with Dementia
Opportunities and Obstacles
Malcolm Goldsmith
Preface by Mary Marshall
ISBN 978 1 85302 406 1

Social Work and Dementia
Good Practice and Care Management
Margaret Anne Tibbs
Foreword by Murna Downs
ISBN 978 1 85302 904 2

The Perspectives of People with Dementia
Research Methods and Motivations
Edited by Heather Wilkinson
ISBN 978 1 84310 001 0

Creative Writing in Health and Social Care
Edited by Fiona Sampson
Foreword by Christina Patterson
ISBN 978 1 84310 136 9

Ageing, Spirituality and Well-being
Edited by Albert Jewell
ISBN 978 1 84310 167 3

Dementia and Social Inclusion

Marginalised Groups and Marginalised Areas of Dementia Research, Care and Practice

*Edited by Anthea Innes, Carole Archibald
and Charlie Murphy*

Jessica Kingsley Publishers
London and Philadelphia

First published in 2004
by Jessica Kingsley Publishers
116 Pentonville Road
London N1 9JB, UK
and
400 Market Street, Suite 400
Philadelphia, PA 19106, USA

www.jkp.com

Library of Congress Cataloging in Publication Data
Dementia and social inclusion : marginalised groups and marginalised areas of dementia
research, care and practice / edited by Anthea Innes, Carole Archibald and Charlie
Murphy.
        p. cm.
    Includes bibliographical references and index.
    ISBN 1-84310-174-2 (pbk.)
1. Dementia--Patients--Care. 2. Dementia--Patients--Services for. I. Innes, Anthea. II.
Archibald, Carole. III. Murphy, Charlie, 1960-
    RC521.D45335 2004
    616.8'3--dc22

                                                                        2004010960

British Library Cataloguing in Publication Data
A CIP catalogue record for this book is available from the British Library

ISBN 978 1 84310 174 1

Printed and Bound in Great Britain by
Athenaeum Press, Gateshead, Tyne and Wear

For Colin Bell, an inspirational social scientist and mentor

Acknowledgements

Thanks to the British Academy and Janssen-Cilag for their sponsorship of the symposium that led to the book. In addition there are three people who in particular have influenced the production of this book. The first is the late Colin Bell who helped nurture the initial idea for this book, perhaps without realising he did so. We would like to thank Alison Bowes for overseeing the editing process of the book during Anthea Innes' maternity leave and Jennifer Gordon for her excellent secretarial support.

Editors' Note

Names and personal details of the subjects of the case studies in this book have been changed to protect the identity of those involved.

Contents

Introduction

*Anthea Innes, Carole Archibald
and Charlie Murphy*

It is widely recognised that dementia as a field of study has grown in popularity in the last 30 years creating an exciting time of opportunity for further theorising dementia and improving practice. Since the 1970s there have been shifts from dementia being the preserve of medics and psychologists to an ever-growing interest in the topic from within the social sciences (Innes 2002) and this is reflected in the terminology used. This has changed from the 'sufferer' of dementia, their families and professional carers to the person with dementia, informal carers and formal carers who often do not have professional qualifications (Bryden 2002; Downs 2000).

The introduction of a new language to discuss dementia does not necessarily mean that changes will have occurred in practice and service development. Despite the progress that has undoubtedly been made in dementia there remain areas that have been largely overlooked. This indicates that within the study of dementia there is a tendency to relegate certain issues, which are often difficult and challenging, to the margins of academic and professional discourses. There are parallels here with how the study of dementia itself was, and perhaps still is, perceived to be difficult and challenging.

Throughout the book a range of topics highlighting issues which have been marginalised within dementia research, care or practice are addressed. For example, people with dementia from minority ethnic groups have been overlooked; the sexuality of people with dementia has been perceived as a taboo topic, as has faecal incontinence. The lives of people with dementia in remote and rural communities have tended to be ignored in favour of an exploration of experiences of people in urban areas. The final phase of the spectrum of dementia care – palliative care – is a phase of care that has scarcely been addressed by researchers and academics. This book sets out to bring topics such as these to the fore so that both dementia and dementia care may be theorised and understood in its entirety as opposed to groups and topics that have been more attractive to those commissioning research and services.

The growing body of work in the dementia care field – reflected in specialist journals, books and education programmes – indicates the growing interest in dementia from academic and professional communities. Unfortunately this has yet to mature to a point of a truly inclusive agenda. This book therefore has an ambitious vision of beginning to move discussion of certain marginalised areas of dementia research, policy and practice on from their neglected, Cinderella status to one of mainstreaming and inclusion.

The concept of social inclusion, which is bringing many traditionally marginalised groups into the mainstream of policy, research and practice, has received little attention, with a few exceptions, in the field of dementia studies. Throughout this book we seek to explore and challenge the reasons behind the neglect or marginalisation of certain issues within the field of dementia care. It is hoped that the reader of this book will be stimulated to think beyond the stereotyping that occurs for this group of people that has resulted in the marginalisation and exclusion within both society and academia.

Throughout the chapters of this book we look at the barriers and provide arguments and a rationale for the inclusion of people with dementia in these neglected areas within dementia studies. The key challenge for the future of dementia care is to look at how we can engage with notions of social inclusion, citizenship and the rights of people with dementia. This book does not claim to have the answers to this question but it is hoped that it will go some way in contributing to the debates on mainstreaming all aspects of dementia care rather than marginalising them as 'special' or 'different'.

The chapters in this book are drawn in part from an international symposium in November 2002 at the University of Stirling. The title of this symposium was 'Dementia: an inclusive future? Marginalised groups and marginalised areas of dementia care, research and practice'. The aim of the symposium was to draw attention to marginalised areas of service development, theory and research. Academia has tended to overlook dementia, resulting in an under-theorised area of work. Certain values have also guided the development of this book, with ways to include people with dementia throughout the research process being suggested. The necessity of acknowledging the personhood of all people with dementia – regardless of, for example, their ethnicity, religious beliefs, sexuality or other sources of multiple oppressions – features throughout the book. The vision of an inclusive process where people with dementia retain citizenship within society and are valued members of communities is also a recurrent theme of the book.

Part 1 of the book begins with a consideration of social changes occurring in the last two decades and the impact these have had on the development of dementia research, care and practice. The opening chapter by Colin Bell highlights that older people and people with dementia have not traditionally been included in many studies of community. He argues that this reflects a widespread ageism throughout society and academia. He suggests that for people with dementia to be included in our understandings of community and communion, relationships between older people and relationships between people with dementia and those who do not have dementia need to be further explored. The book continues with a discussion by Anthea Innes and Kirsty Sherlock about dementia in rural Scottish communities. This chapter is an initial attempt to explore the lives of people with dementia in rural Scotland through a specific examination of experiences of service provision in remote and rural communities in Scotland. Rural communities tend to be ageing communities; however, much dementia research has focused on more populated urban areas to the extent that very little is known about living with dementia in rural areas. The general problems experienced by older people and people with dementia tend to be exacerbated in rural areas, highlighting the need for flexible service provision.

The main focus of care in the community is that of keeping people in their own homes. Family carers are central to this policy but so too are home care workers. Although service provision in institutions has received much attention, explorations of services designed to help maintain people with dementia in their own homes are few. Home care in particular has been the subject of much change in the last ten years with more intimate care being provided than previously and people with greater needs being targeted. The final chapter in Part 1 by Noni Cobban discusses how to improve home care services for people with dementia. This chapter addresses the problems that staff, who are often untrained and poorly supported, face in delivering home care to people with dementia. In line with the ethos of this book it offers recommendations for developing the support and training needs of home carers to enable them to continue to deliver person-centred care.

There have been to date some socio-cultural issues within dementia research that have been subject to limited academic scrutiny. Part 2 explores some of these socio-cultural issues, namely ethnicity and spirituality, dying with dementia and sexuality. Each chapter in this part summarises the recent interest in these otherwise marginalised topics, and discusses aspects that remain overlooked but that are worthy of future attention. The first chapter in Part 2 by Peggye Dilworth-Anderson is an exploration of the role of spirituality and religion in the care of people with dementia as reported by African Americans. Distinguishing between religion and spirituality this chapter does two things: it first looks at ethnicity, and second addresses religion and spirituality. Peggye Dilworth-Anderson provides a theoretical overview, employs the findings from a large empirical study and discusses the relevant literature, to explore the role that both spirituality and religiosity play in helping African American caregivers in their caregiving role.

Palliative care is at the final point on the spectrum of dementia care and as such it is perhaps unsurprising that it is an area we are only beginning to hear mentioned. As Sylvia Cox and Karen Watchman demonstrate, much can be learnt and applied to dementia from the general palliative care literature. Sex occupies a place similar to death. Both are taboo areas and when dementia is an added component the situation is made worse. Foucault (1979) argued that people understood sexuality through discourses or sets of knowledges that society makes available to them. Out of strategies of normalisation emerges a sense of what sexuality is and what it should be. For many this does not include older people and specifically people with dementia. Sexuality has been neglected in both research, policy and practice. Carole Archibald's chapter exploring sexuality in residential homes concludes this part of the book. In both the literature and in her empirical work, Carole Archibald looks at how both dementia and sexuality are constructed and the influence this has on staff response to residents' expression of sexuality.

Marginalised dementia care issues are the focus of Part 3. A discussion by Christian Müller-Hergl of the often 'taboo' topic of faecal continence opens this part of the book. Through a series of vignettes this chapter challenges the reader to consider what communication might be taking place in certain episodes of incontinence, while simultaneously exploring the power relationships within long-stay care and particularly with respect to intimate physical care. Errollyn Bruce discusses the findings of empirical work undertaken by herself and colleagues in residential care homes and applies an inverse care law (Brooker *et al.* 1998) to explore how three common routes to social inclusion occur. This provides a fascinating and original take on people with dementia in residential care. Case material from a longitudinal study is used to illustrate that as dementia becomes more advanced, the likelihood of appropriate care for emotional, physical, occupational, spiritual and social needs decreases. Part 3 concludes with a discussion from Jill Manthorpe of risk taking and dementia care. Although risk taking has a long history and is not necessarily perceived as a marginalised topic there is still a tendency to avoid and protect people with dementia from taking risks. This chapter sets out the context and future directions for this area of care practice.

Part 4 of the book draws attention to the importance of continuing to develop communication with people with dementia. Communicating with people with dementia is a central aspect of an inclusive research agenda, developing appropriate services and central to acknowledging the personhood of individuals with dementia. The ways in which the words of people with dementia are represented by researchers and practitioners and the potential to overlook the views of individuals who may be marginalised due to communication difficulties are both addressed in this part of the book. Rik Cheston draws on his work with people with dementia in psychotherapy groups to demonstrate how people with dementia come to terms with their dementia. In a very personal account he challenges any notions of a correct response with a specific contrast between those who respond as survivors and those who react as victims. The potential of support groups for people with dementia is manifested throughout this chapter. Gillian McColgan's chapter draws on her research with people with dementia in residential homes and demonstrates the ability of people with dementia to be research informants in their own right while re-presenting their experiences of dementia and life in a nursing home. The growing recognition of the arts as a form of communication provides the basis for the final chapter in this part, written by Claire Craig, with a postscript by John Killick. The chapter expands upon the role of the arts in reinforcement of identity and in self-expression, encouraging the reader to see the arts as integral to the environment for people with dementia and not as a luxury adjunct.

Part 5, the concluding part of the book, brings together the theoretical and applied aspects of dementia research. Medical perspectives have long dominated dementia discourses. Perhaps the principal benefit of such a focus has been the emergence of anti-dementia drugs which have had the effect of 'holding' disease progression (Anand, Messina and Hartman 2000). The chapter by Michael Bradbury, Clive Ballard and Andrew Fairbairn highlights the dominant focus of medical interests while pointing out areas within medical disciplines that have been marginalised. These authors explore such issues as hypertension and dementia, and diabetes and dementia, and look at an area that is now starting to attract increasing attention, that of vascular dementia. John Bond, Lynne Corner and Ruth Graham's chapter demonstrates that social gerontology and social science can provide insights into the process of including people with dementia in the future. Social science perspectives are slowly developing in dementia research. Wendy Hulko's chapter is an example of ongoing research that draws on a range of social science theory to the study of class, race and gender oppressions experienced by people with dementia.

The final chapter of the book by Caroline Cantley and Alison Bowes points the way to a more inclusive future in relation to values, service development, and theory and research. Cantley and Bowes argue that the values of maintaining personhood, valuing the relationships of people with dementia with others and recognising their rights as citizens are central to inclusive processes. For service development to be inclusive, services need to be responsive to individual needs; this requires innovative working practices and an engagement with the centrality of social relationships to providing person-centred services. For people with dementia to receive person-centred services requires a greater investment in staff.

The contributors to this book discuss ways to involve people with dementia in the research process and there are also reports from empirical work highlighting exclusionary processes; therefore this book is a contribution to filling some of the gaps in current knowledge. The key issues for the future identified by Cantley and Bowes relate to the need for an exploration of difference and commonality in the experience of dementia with the goal of learning from this process to promote inclusion of all people with dementia. Service specialisation, policy development, advocacy and collective action are given as examples of taking dementia towards a more inclusive future. This book is a small stepping stone to understanding how academics, policy makers and practitioners can work with the challenge of obtaining a future of social inclusion for people with dementia.

References

Anand, R., Messina, J. and Hartman, R. (2000) 'Dose response effect of Rivistigmine in the treatment of Alzheimer's disease.' *International Journal of Geriatric Psychopharmacology 2*, 68–72.

Brooker, D., Foster, N., Banner, A., Payne, M. and Jackson, L. (1998) 'The efficacy of dementia care mapping as an audit tool: report of a 3-year British MHS evaluation.' *Ageing and Mental Health 2*, 1, 60–70.

Bryden, C. (2002) 'A person centred approach to counselling, psychotherapy and rehabilitation of people diagnosed with dementia in the early stages.' *Dementia: The International Journal of Social Research and Practice 1*, 2, 141–156.

Downs, M. (2000) 'Dementia in a social-cultural context: an idea whose time has come.'
    Ageing and Society 20, 3, 369–373.

Foucault, M. (1979) *The History of Sexuality*, Volume 1. London: Penguin.

Innes, A. (2002) 'The social and political context of formal dementia care provision.'
    Ageing and Society 22, 4, 483–500.

PART 1
Dementia and Social Change

CHAPTER 1

Dementia and Social Change: Views from a Sociologist of the Community

Colin Bell

Where we have come from

The person and character of Peter Townsend casts a long shadow over the sociology of old age in Britain and beyond. Ever since *The Family Life of Old People* (Townsend 1957) was published, it should have been impossible to ignore not just older persons' family life but their position in the community as well. It is with that latter point that I am immediately concerned here. Townsend's book was of course produced from the famous Institute of Community Studies and is very much in the style of its founders, Michael Young and Peter Willmott. Its location was the same too – Bethnal Green in working class East London. Forever, there will be a debate about just how far we can extrapolate from there to the rest of society – to different places and to different classes. I would add, too, to different times. How much has changed over the half-century since through, say, rehousing, geographical and social mobility, affluence and occupational change, let alone transformation through social policies of the welfare state? Nevertheless, there are many themes in this pioneering enquiry that are still with us and, I will argue here, remain unresolved and essentially contested. Our understanding and conceptualisation, indeed our theorising, remains partial.

Townsend showed just how *near* many of these older people lived to their families. Like others at the Institute of Community Studies, he 'rediscovered' the extended family and in particular emphasised the importance, emotionally and structurally, of the mother–married daughter 'tie'. He placed particular emphasis on his samples' 'contacts' – and not simply on their number (the 'how many' question) but also on their quality. He shows just how devastating the loss of a daughter, often through geographical mobility but *in extremis* through death, was for older people. But he does take 'community' seriously and I want to explore that conceptual minefield a little more closely.

Community, as Townsend knows, is much more than an idea. But it is an idea. It is an ideology too. All this has made it one of the trickiest of sociological concepts.[1]

I have argued before (Bell and Newby 1978) that when feelings about social relationships in a locality (or even an organisation I would now say) are involved we could use the term 'communion' rather than community.

But following Townsend, 'community' need not be so tricky! Let us focus not so much on place but on social relationships. And keep those separate. Much confusion has been caused by locating particular social relationships in particular places. Even more has been caused by giving causal force to place onto social relationships and viewing them through nostalgia-tinted glasses! That allows the forces of industrialisation and its associated urbanisation to be forever causing community to be changed, or even destroyed. This perspective of course allowed community, with extended family relationships at its core, to be 'rediscovered' by all the colleagues at the Institute of Community Studies. The very best of these studies, *Family and Social Change* (Rosser and Harris 1965), does show that their findings could hold true in a very different urban area, Swansea. That book, through its marvellous opening case study of the 'Hughes family, Morriston', also explores the comparatively shallow historical and generational depth that some of today's patterns actually have.

What does come out of Townsend's pioneering work is an enduring concern with 'isolation' and with 'loneliness'. I want to argue this is still a useful approach and can help to make the concept of community less tricky. Published in the same year was *Family and Social Network* (Bott 1957). I want to adapt Elizabeth Bott's insights into the social relationships of what she calls ordinary urban families and build upon Townsend's findings.

'Isolation' can be embedded in notions of the 'structure' of social relations. The Institute of Community Studies usually counted 'contacts' – how many in the last week and so on. Bott moved on and related that to the 'close knittedness', or otherwise, of social networks. This can be (over) simply understood as finding out how many of your contacts know each other – often though this turns out to be how many and what proportion of these relationships are, in reality, kin. Many in Townsend's samples were living in close-knit networks – those that were not, who had fewer contacts, turn out to be 'isolated' in Townsend's terms.

This though tells us little about the quality or the content of these relationships. We need a different way of understanding this. If 'knittedness' (or density) is about the structure of social relationships, maybe we should speak of 'plexity' with regard to the content of relationship. Plexity varies from the *uniplex* (famously in the sociological literature the taxi-driver and his fare), through *simplex* to the *complex* (e.g. the complexity of, say, mother–married daughter ties). Those who do not have complex relationships in Townsend's study turn out to be 'lonely' in his terms.

Community then may be understood through such an approach. As usually, and in our culture popularly, understood, 'communities' exhibit dense structures – are close knit, and involve complex social relationships. Many social processes of advanced industrial societies – for instance social and geographical mobility – will be seen as eroding these dense structures of complex relationships, of changing and usually damaging community. But we should not get over-excited here, nor exaggerate changes. *Social Trends 2003* (National Statistics 2003) reports from excellent data sets that 61 per cent of grandparents still see their grandchildren *at least* once a week.

So, simply, what we have here is a powerful tradition that has focused on older people's relationships – charting relative isolation (which should now be seen in terms of the *structure* of social relationships) and loneliness (which should now be seen in terms of the *content* of social relationships). Many have been concerned with the implications of the structure and content of social relationships for the survival, health and illness of older people. A very fine example of this tradition is *Old and Cold: Hypothermia and Social Policy* (Wicks 1978), which shows clearly how the threat of death from hypothermia was closely related to isolation and loneliness, to the structure and content of social relationships. This is a better way sociologically than simply speaking of community and makes empirical exploration, operationalisation as it were, so much more possible.

Where we are now

Before turning the direction of our attention round I want just to point out that in our kind of societies community *has* in some senses become placeless (whereas in the past it was always understood to be somewhere). Long-lasting, close-knit networks of complex relationships – exerting social control and feelings of belonging that support identity and our feelings and notions of selfhood and our very being – are less now a characteristic of Bethnal Green than of occupational and professional 'communities'. That dementia as a field is professionalising, typified by this book, I take to be very significant.

The older sociological tradition though has been about their (older persons') relationships. I want to argue that in this field, as in so many others (some of which I will turn to shortly), it is sociologically and politically productive to turn the focus round. For an early reflective account and series of arguments in this direction see my 'Studying the locally powerful' in *Inside the Whale* (Bell and Encel 1978). I am silent there on older people – and in this am typical of much social science. What about *our* relationships with older people: what about those *structures* and *contents*?

This is similar to but more overtly political in many ways than the ideas that can be derived from Norbert Elias' figurational sociology. He himself was the author of a particularly inspirational and wise book: *The Loneliness of the Dying* (Elias 1985). Elias (p.172) is so clear that the experience of ageing people cannot be understood 'unless we realise that the process of ageing openly brings about a fundamental change in a person's position in society, and so in his or her whole relationships to other people'. The use of the word 'whole' should strike chords with contemporary colleagues working on issues of dementia care. Elias is painfully articulate on the *emotional* loneliness of the dying and the special form of the relationships of people to the dying in more developed societies.

He also is the author of a community study, *The Established and the Outsiders* (Elias and Scotson 1965), which I believe to be very relevant to our themes. He noted how the 'established' – in this case families in a suburban housing development – were always judged by their very best people and the 'outsiders' by their worst. This had little to do with numbers and lots to do with culture and has remarkable continuities. For the non-old – the rest of us as it were – we are the established and they are the outsiders. And we are judgemental.

The gains that have been made recently in our understanding of racism and sexism, of discriminatory actions around disability or sexual orientation, have not come from studying black people, women, the physically challenged or the gay. Attention should be, and has been, shifted from the victim, as it were, to the powerful. Racism may have awful implications for black people but to understand the embedded nature of institutionalised racism we had better study the actions, activities, practices and ideologies of the powerful, and usually white and usually men. That is now clearly understood, particularly in a post-MacPherson (1999) world in the UK and reflected remarkably in the recent Race Relations Amendment Act of 2000.

The most productive sociological research programme that could be proposed now on older people would be to turn the focus 'from them to us' – to look, as I said, at our relationships with them. This must remain, I'm sorry to say, essentially speculative. I, at least, know of hardly any work that has turned its sociological attention round in this way, let alone capturing the worldview of those with dementia. If a start has been made at all it is with a group of not very powerful people – care workers, who did of course at least figure in another pioneering Townsend work: *The Last Refuge* (Townsend 1972). This, though it takes us far from concern about community, does introduce another powerful (and powerfully confused) notion: emotional labour. When Arlie Hochschild (1983) popularised this term she was building on an empirical study of air hostesses but connecting to what a lot of women do *at work*, as well as *at home*. 'Emotional labour' is a fine example of the complexity of social relationships in the terms that were introduced earlier. The sociology of emotions is relatively underdeveloped but see Veronica James and Jonathan Gabe's *Health and the Sociology of Emotions* (1996). James' work in hospices is very relevant to the themes of this book (James 1989, 1993). See too Geraldine Lee Treweek's 'Emotion work in care assistant work' (1996) which emphasises the close links between emotional work, power and the need to create order. Given that it is far from clear that much, or any, of emotional labour is directly paid for in employment contracts there are many issues here. (I am reminded sharply here about the additionality of emotional labour and welfare work that my university gets from its cleaning staff through their relationships with students in halls of residences – which we'd never get if that service was contracted out.)

Too great an emphasis on care workers – important though that emphasis is – would almost keep us too close to older people, especially in institutions and facilities. What about 'out there', the wider community, however understood? There isn't time or space to elaborate here but drivers of change include:

- demographics
- changing pace of generations
- revolutions in gender relations
- household composition
- communication revolutions.

To that we could add this decade's cliché: globalisation, or worldwide labour markets at many levels – from asylum seekers and economic immigrants to global geographical mobility through multinational companies.

So simply: we do have to take on the issues around an ageing population. Life expectancy, outside Africa, is increasing world-wide, particularly in societies like ours. There is a tremendous increase now in the number of men living into their 80s. We know that, even in recent months, there have been increasingly panicky political and fiscal problems over pensions. The burden. The burden! All the sharper too with continuing stock market decline – let alone war. There will need to be an even livelier political economy of old age. 'Dependency ratios', so called, are being calculated with increasing alarm. *Social Trends 2003* reports a 51 per cent increase (9.4 million) of people aged 65 or over since 1961 – and 1.1 million over 85 which is three times as many as in 1961. Some of these demographics are behind the concerns of this book in that many will argue that increasing amounts (if not prevalence) of dementia or intellectual impairment along with other 'giants of gerontology' – immobility, incontinence and instability – seen in our societies are a direct consequence of many people living longer. This is what some have called 'the survival of the unfittest'. These four 'disabilities' have, as is well known, four common properties – they have multiple causes, they destroy independence, there is no simple treatment (hence the failure of the so-called 'medical model') and they need human helpers.

But their daughters now are in employment for increasing periods of their lives (and their mother, their children's grandmother, is also increasingly out at work too) and so are unavailable, even if they remain unusually physically close, for emotional and physical care. These are now so-called 'beanpole families' – those with fewer children and multiple older generations. Despite all this increase in employment (and most of the increase in the single number of jobs has been in female employment) nobody is earning enough to pay for care. Re-mortgaging, de-mortgaging and destroying expected domestic inheritances is not meeting the need. And the welfare state and its universalistic principles are being rolled back in the face of a low tax economy and a weakened local state. The same *Social Trends 2003* reports that 63 per cent of the British public think that it is the government's responsibility to provide a decent standard of living for the old.

Many households are simply too poor to pay for care – many are female headed and there is a significant growth in the number of people living alone through their 30s and thereafter.

Where we might go

Some of these social changes have led some to make comments on the erosion of *civil society*, and diminishing *social capital*. Tremendously influential here is Robert Putman's *Bowling Alone* (Putman 2000) – indeed this Harvard political scientist has given seminars at Number Ten even!

Bowling alone is more than an elaborate metaphor. Americans used to bowl together, in clubs and leagues; now they bowl alone. The subtitle of his book is *The Collapse and Revival of American Community*. Putman assembles staggeringly impressive sets of (often longitudinal) data that shows not only do they bowl alone, if at all, but they don't go to PTAs, boy scouts, churches even as much as they did. They are just not out and about together like they were once upon a time in America. He displays the ominous implications of this for local charitable and voluntary activity. He considers too whether informal activity – ordinary sociability – has increased to fill the space once occupied by more formal activity. As far as he can tell, again with goodish data, it has not. Why is this happening? – and the evidence does impress that it really is.

He takes a list of causes – not unlike mine, above (which indeed was partially drawn from his) – and through very sophisticated statistical manipulation of his excellent data set shows that it does have (a little) to do with being 'time poor' through both adults working long hours, weeks and years and travelling too far to work because of suburbanisation and exurbanisation. He also shows the damaging amount of time taken up by watching television (now surfing the Internet I guess) – but is this a cause or consequence of something else?

Here there is controversy and debate. Are we seeing major cultural change – away from community and caring and concern and voluntary activity towards isolation, cash nexus household focus? And if we go out, we bowl alone (of course playing computer games merely simulates bowling alone).

Putman points to issues about intergenerational change but doesn't elaborate the implications for older people. But the great 'long civic generation' of middle generation, middlemass of middle America seems now to have acquired great incapacity socially. There are issues that could be explored about incapacity physically too and its implications for later life health – we might live longer, as I asked in the last section, but will we be well?

Putman does take on the communication revolution to return to earlier themes, but does not say much about the implications for contact and the content of social relationships. Families might have moved away but do they telephone and email? Modern communications are, naturally enough, virtually unmentioned in Townsend. By the 1960s when I was doing the work on *Middle Class Families* (Bell 1968) the telephone *was* important for contact but it didn't stop the geographically mobile feeling lonely and socially impoverished. Putman, unlike some utopians, does *not* see the communication revolution leading to the rebuilding of *social capital*.

All this is controversial – not least as to whether *Bowling Alone* (Putman 2000) is all too American and doesn't apply here. But it does raise important issues about local voluntary activity, about caring and concern and the charitable urge and the gift relationship being replaced by Live Aid followed by compassion fatigue. Putman has reinvigorated the rather tired debate about community and society. It is as if Margaret Thatcher *was* right, but about America! There is no such thing as society – just people who bowl alone. There are real issues here about alienation and lack of meaning in people's lives that are frankly pessimistic.

Putman's thesis has recently been reviewed for Britain by Peter A. Hall (1999) and he considers the evidence from both formal organisations and as well as the direct concerns of this chapter of 'a more diffused set of social relations, whether rooted in the family, community, class structure or associational life' (p.417), 'notably the kind of face to face relations of relative equality associated with participation in common endeavours, whether recreational, social, service orientated or political' (p.418). In line with the general Putman thesis, the premise is that the social networks generated by such patterns of sociability constitute important forms of 'social capital' in, as Hall says, 'the sense that they increase the trust that individuals feel towards others and enhance their capacity to join together in collective action to resolve common problems or to ensure that governments address such problems' (p.418).

But in contrast to the USA, Hall finds *no* equivalent erosion in Britain, no undermining of the capacity for generalised reciprocity. The voluntary sector in Britain is extensive and vibrant. Time budget data contradicts suggestions that the British have become increasingly privatised. Instead, even a conservative interpretation would suggest that there has been some expansion in informal sociability over the last 40 years (p.427). This is difficult to explain, for it seems that although levels of community involvement measured by associational membership, charitable endeavour and informal sociability appear to have declined in the United States, they have remained resilient in Britain. Changes in female labour-force participation rates, working time and family status don't seem to have had the same impact in Britain. Nor does the telly!

Hall sees the causes as lying first in the educational revolution – the vast expansion of secondary and post-secondary education since the time, for instance, of Townsend's first book. Every additional year of education increases the propensity of an individual to become involved in community affairs, whether by joining an association or providing voluntary work for the community. Second, he highlights the impact of changes in the British class structure – especially the growth in the size of the middle class. Goldthorpe (1987) describes the essential change as the growth of an increasingly substantial 'service class'. And there is strong evidence that the upwardly mobile have adopted the sociability patterns of the class into which they have moved. And third there is the effect of government policy – British governments not only have made substantial efforts to ensure that voluntary activity flourishes, they have also adopted an approach to social policy that makes extensive use of volunteers, alongside professionals, for the delivery of social services. Perhaps this is nowhere more true than of services to older people. These are then reasons to be much more optimistic about Britain. As Hall powerfully concludes:

> …the willingness to trust others is ultimately related to what sociologists often term the character of social integration in a society, understood in the way in which people relate to others and their understanding of their own role in society. There are many indications that the character of social integration shifted in Britain during the post-war decades, and some features of that shift may have affected levels of social change. (Hall 1999, p.446)

Conclusion

I do think that it is important to get some of these ideas on the agenda before taking on dementia. I do know too that they raise as many questions as they resolve. But they are good questions that may breathe new life into old but important arguments about the relationship between ourselves and society – indeed about the very nature of community. Let's talk about our relationships both with each other and with older people across the generations. One of the great ideas around in this field is the notion of whole personhood – seeing in this case the whole person, not just a bearer of dementia. That would, of course, include exploring all social relationships including our own with that person. In part – maybe in the most important part – this is to conclude by making statements about the need to reconnect, in itself the source of authenticity in our social relationships. That is the direction towards which we should strive and which would give all our lives more meaning. As one fine example of this I'd like to leave you with the moving piece to be found at the end of Simone de Beauvoir's (1983) farewell to Jean-Paul Sartre:

Should I have not warned Sartre of the imminence of death?... If he had been more exactly aware of the threat that hung over him, it would have darkened his last years without doing any good...my silence does not separate us.

His death does separate us. My death will not bring us together again. That is how things are. It is in itself splendid that we were able to live our lives in harmony for so long. (pp.26–7)

This should be a source of optimism because even if we don't make our lives in circumstances of our own choosing we can still make them. After all the Iris Murdoch Building for Dementia Care at the University of Stirling did get built. It is an unexpected monument to the continuing, even growing, strength of British civil society and the sheer power of community and communion today.

Note

1   For an overview that embeds community in the historical and theoretical sociological tradition see Robert Nisbet's incomparable *The Sociological Tradition* (Nisbet 1966) and for an overview that centres on that tradition's empirical achievements in the British Isles and North America see my juvenile work, *Community Studies* (Bell and Newby 1971).

References

Bell, C. (1968) *Middle Class Families*. London: Routledge.

Bell, C. and Encel, S. (eds) (1978) *Inside the Whale*. Sydney and Oxford: Pergamon.

Bell, C. and Newby, H. (1971) *Community Studies*. London: Allen and Unwin.

Bell, C. and Newby, H. (1978) 'Community, communion, class and community action: the social sources of the new urban politics.' In D.T. Herbert and R.J. Johnson (eds) *Social Areas in Cities*. Chichester: Wiley.

Bott, E. (1957) *Family and Social Network*. London: Tavistock.

de Beauvoir, S. (1983) *Adieux: A Farewell to Sartre*. Harmondsworth: Penguin.

Elias, N. (1985) *The Loneliness of the Dying*. Oxford: Blackwell.

Elias, N. and Scotson, J.L. (1965) *The Established and the Outsiders*. London: Cass.

Goldthorpe, J. (1987) *Social Mobility and Class Structure in Modern Britain*. Oxford: Clarendon.

Hall, P.A. (1999) 'Social capital in Britain.' *British Journal of Political Science 29*, 417–461.

Hochschild, A. (1983) *The Managed Heart: The Commercialisation of Human Feeling*. Berkeley: University of California.

James, N. (1989) 'Emotional labour: skill and work in the social regulation of feelings.' *Sociological Review 37*, 15–42.

James, N. (1993) 'Divisions of emotional labour: disclosure and cancer.' In S. Fineman (ed) *Emotion in Organization*. London: Sage.

James, V. and Gabe, J. (1996) *Health and the Sociology of Emotions*. Oxford: Blackwell.

MacPherson, W. (1999) *The Stephen Lawrence Inquiry*. London: HMSO.

National Statistics (2003) *Social Trends 2003* C. Summerfield and P. Babb (eds) London: The Stationary Office.

Nisbet, R. (1966) *The Sociological Tradition*. London: Heinemann.

Putman, R.D. (2000) *Bowling Alone: The Collapse and Revival of American Community*. New York: Simon and Schuster.

Rosser, C. and Harris, C.C. (1965) *Family and Social Change*. London: Routledge.

Townsend, P. (1957) *The Family Life of Old People*. Harmondsworth: Penguin.

Townsend, P. (1972) *The Last Refuge*. London: Routledge.

Treweek, G.L. (1996) 'Emotion work in care assistant work.' In N. James and J. Gabe (eds) *Health and the Sociology of Emotions*. Oxford: Blackwell.

Wicks, M. (1978) *Old and Cold: Hypothermia and Social Policy*. Oxford: Heinemann.

CHAPTER 2

Rural Communities

Anthea Innes and Kirsty Sherlock

Introduction

This chapter is based on research with service providers, people with dementia (PWD) and their informal carers working and living in remote and rural areas of Scotland.

The key aim of the Scottish research was to explore the availability and accessibility of services for people with dementia and their carers from the viewpoints of:

1. service providers

2. people with dementia

3. the informal carers of people with dementia.

By giving voice to this group of under-researched service providers and service users, we enabled these groups to outline not only their experiences of provision but also their definition of gaps and limitations in services provided.

This chapter begins by outlining why a research focus on remote and rural Scotland is required, why it is important to include the views of people with dementia and the approach adopted in our research study. We then go on to discuss our research findings relating to service provision for people with dementia and their carers in remote and rural Scotland. These findings cover availability, accessibility, gaps, innovations, problems and opportunities. We conclude with a brief discussion about the future of dementia service provision in remote and rural Scotland.

Background

Why we need a research focus on remote and rural Scotland

Rural communities' experience of dementia care is an area of relative neglect globally. What is known about dementia in rural areas is largely based on research conducted outwith Scotland. For example, research has been conducted in Scandinavia (Sjobeck and Isacsson 1994), North America (Camicioli *et al.* 2000) and Australia (O'Reilly and Strong 1997), with research in the United Kingdom largely limited to North Wales (Wenger 2001) and small studies in specific areas of rural England (Le Mesurier and Duncan 2000) or counties in Northern Ireland (Gilmour 2002). Although the needs of rural communities in Scotland were identified as an area requiring development in the late 1990s (Dementia Services Development Centre 1998) the first survey of service providers in remote and rural areas throughout Scotland was only conducted in 2002 (Innes *et al.* 2002). In rural Scotland there is a marked lack of information about the experiences of people with dementia and their carers' experience and views on service provision. This contrasts with other countries where the prevalence of dementia in rural areas (Camicioli *et al.* 2000; Gilmour, Gibson and Campbell 2003), the experiences of carers (e.g. O'Reilly and Strong 1997) and evaluations of innovative measures to provide services for people with dementia and their carers (e.g. Paul, Johnson and Cranston 2000) have received researchers' attention. A number of myths are said to surround older people living in rural areas – that these people have strong family support networks; that they belong to an integrated community; that they have better health; and that they live in pleasant conditions, resulting in a low demand for services (Wenger 2001). One study in Sweden suggests that older people with dementia in rural areas use services more than those who do not have dementia (Sjobeck and Isacsson 1994). There is, however, no evidence to support or reject these assumptions in relation to dementia in Scotland. Recent work carried out in relation to quality of services in rural Scotland has included reference to the generic older population's views (Hope, Anderson and Sawyer 2000) or health service provision in general and older people's services in particular (Shucksmith and Murphy 1999). Surveys have examined local community care needs and services available (West Highland Project 1992). However, such work does not provide information on dementia specifically nor use of health and social care services for carers and people with dementia. Individual local authorities may have assessed the need for services in their area for people with dementia.[1] This does not appear to be the norm, however, and does not tell us of services available across sectors, nor the experiences of the users of available services, both carers and people with dementia.

There may be parallels in Scotland with findings of research in other countries. However, every country has a specific social, political and economic context. Demographic factors (below) in Scotland demonstrate that research was also required in Scotland:

- the projected increase in the number of older people in Scotland in the next two decades (Armstrong 2002)

- in addition, older people comprise a large proportion of population in remote and rural areas of Scotland due to:

  - out-migration of younger people

  - in-migration of retired older people to rural areas

  - people living longer.

Also dementia research in other countries did not, in the main, seek to include the views of people with dementia themselves.

The importance of including the perspectives of persons with dementia

Including the views of persons with dementia was a central feature of the research. This approach is grounded in the perspective that it is possible and desirable to hear the voice of people with dementia (Goldsmith 1996; Nolan *et al.* 2002; Wilkinson 2002) on all issues relating to their care and quality of life (Innes and Capstick 2001; Kitwood 1997).

It is interesting to note that in our research around three-quarters of service provider organisations consulted with other service providers (78%) and with older people (74%) who use services. Notably, only 54 per cent of services consult with older people with dementia. The same number of carers were consulted in developing services whether they were carers of older people or people with dementia (66%). Also, 79 per cent of service providers consulted with carers of people with dementia about dementia services but did not consult with the person with dementia. Therefore, seeking the views of those who used the services was a crucial dimension to this research and is based on the growing body of work confirming that it is possible to hear the views of people with dementia by using appropriate techniques (Cook 2002; Corner 2002; Proctor 2001). In our research we successfully recruited and obtained consent from 17 people with dementia. Each person participated in a face-to-face semi-structured interview.

Including the voices of those who live in dispersed remote communities can also pose challenges for researchers, in terms of recruiting a sample and implementing the data collection, due to dispersed target communities and difficulties in maintaining anonymity due to the 'intrusive and controlling' nature of rural community networks (Glendinning *et al.* 2003). A postal survey and follow-up telephone interviews with service providers overcame problems of distance, as did a telephone focus group with carers who also found it difficult to leave the person they cared for.

Methods

The discussion that follows is based on data collected from:

- a postal survey of 193 service providers from voluntary, statutory and private sectors (46% response rate)
- follow-up telephone interviews with 11 service providers selected to include providers from statutory, voluntary and private sectors in different geographical areas
- three focus groups with informal carers (n=14)
- face-to-face semi-structured interviews with informal carers (n=17, none of whom participated in a focus group)
- face-to-face semi-structured interviews with people with dementia (n=16).

Table 2.1 illustrates the geographical spread of our service provider, carer and PWD sample. The regional divisions in the table represent a combination of local authorities, health boards and health trust boundaries to ensure that we included providers, carers and people with dementia from a wide spread of remote and rural locations.

We obtained access to service users through voluntary sector service providers, hence all PWD and carers are those currently using at least one service and all were self-selecting.

Availability of services

The range of services provided varied among respondents in different areas but in the main there were more generic than specialist services. Service providers often found it difficult to identify whether their older people

Table 2.1 Geographical location of respondents						
	Service provider		Carer		PWD	
	N	%	N	%	N	%
Highland	13	26	13**	42	8**	50
Scottish Borders	8	9	2	6.5	–	–
Argyll and Bute	7	8	2	6.5	1	6
Ayrshire	6	7	–	–	2	13
Dumfries and Galloway	6	7	5	16	1	6
Western Isles	6	7	8	26	2	13
Stirling and Clackmannanshire	5	6	–	–	–	–
Angus	3	3	–	–	–	–
Moray/Aberdeenshire	3	3	1	3	1	6
Shetland	3	3	–	–	–	–
Greater Glasgow (outlying accessible rural villages)	2	2	–	–	–	–
Lothians	2	2	–	–	–	–
Orkney	2	2	–	–	–	–
Fife	1	1	–	–	–	–
Perth and Kinross	1	1	–	–	1	6
Not specified	12	14	–	–	–	–
TOTAL	90*	102*	31	100	16	100

*Four respondent organisations provided support in two of the above catchment areas: Ayrshire/Argyll and Bute; Highland/Argyll and Bute; Borders/Lothian; Highland/Shetland.

** Our Highland sample includes our Gaelic-speaking sample (n=8).

services were used by PWD but thought it probable that this would be the case. Therefore, service providers reported on older people services that may or may not be used, or appropriate, for PWD and specialist dementia services. Table 2.2 provides a detailed breakdown of services available for older people and people with dementia.

As can be seen from Table 2.2 day care opportunities were the most frequently reported service for older people and for PWD. Table 2.2 illustrates that there are far fewer specialist services for PWD across almost all types of services. In most cases half the amount of services are specialist as compared to those provided for older people in general. In the majority of cases specialist services for people with dementia accounted for less than 50 per cent of what was available generically for older people.

The most frequently reported service used by the PWD in interviews was day care, as shown in Table 2.3, reflecting service providers' reports that day care was often the main service opportunity available. The most common service that carers reported their relative using was having a formal carer come to the home to provide respite, followed by respite through their relative attending day care.

All service users praised the services they received. The most frequent reasons for PWD's praise referred to interpersonal relationships. An equal number (n=10) enjoyed the company of the service providers (generally formal carers or support workers) and the people they met at day centre or their lunch club.

> Steve: Well just to have a good old chin-wag. And they get through. It's amazing what stuff we do talk about. Even if now and again you get on the wrong track, and it's wait a minute, back track, you've missed a bit somewhere here. It, er, we get on all right. (Taped interview)

Day centres were praised by PWD for being stimulating (n=8), with references to enjoyable pastimes such as crafts or indoor bowling. Carers and PWD (n=6) reported that the PWD enjoyed the meals at their day centre or provided by their home help.

However, ten participants with dementia outlined reasons why they did not like some of the services they were receiving. These included poor relationships with their doctors due to frequent staff turnover (n=4); finding respite or day care disorientating and upsetting (n=3); not connecting with other service users at day centre (n=2); finding attending day care too tiring (n=2); disliking the long trip to day care (n=2); and not enjoying their food (n=1) or the activities (n=1). This list of dislikes highlights how service provision must be individually tailored, as what pleases some users is a source of discontent for others.

Table 2.2 Availability of services

Available services	Number of organisations	
	Generic service for older people	Specialist service for people with dementia
Day care opportunities	28	16
Advice and information	21	9
Residential home	20	10
Short-term break/care	19	9
Personal home care (e.g. bathing)	18	7
Practical home care (e.g. shopping)	17	7
Meals on wheels	17	3
Carer support	15	15
Nursing home	14	5
Advocacy	13	5
Rehabilitation	12	4
Supported housing	12	2
Welfare rights	12	9
Nursing care at home	9	7
Mobile services (e.g. chiropody)	8	3
Outreach support/befriending	8	6
Home repairs/maintenance	7	1
Self-help groups	4	5
Acute medical care	2	0
Assessment	1	1
Community work support	1	1
Talking newspaper	1	0

Table 2.3 Services used by people with dementia and carers

Service	Description	No. (reported by PWD)	No. (reported by carer)
Day care	Collective group who meet regularly for activities and a meal	11	22
Personal support	Visits by social worker, link worker or community psychiatric nurse	9	12
Transport to day centre	Provided by service provider, usually a bus	8	12
Medical advice	Close supportive relationship with local GP or nurse	8	10
Carer comes to house	Formal carer who provides home help and/or respite for informal carer	7	25
Home modifications	Changes to assist with daily living, e.g. rails and chair lifts	4	7
Meals on wheels	Provision of hot meal delivered to their home	4	2
Personal care	Assistance with washing and dressing	2	14
Temporary residential respite	Staying at a residential home for a period of between a weekend and a fortnight to provide respite for informal carer	2	16
Other	Support from optometrist and older people's lunch club	2	2
Residential care	Long-term nursing care	1	9
Support group	Collective of users who work together for self-help	1	14

Benefits for the carer when services were used by the PWD include:

- feeling supported by service providers, who provide both practical advice and emotional support (n=25)
- appreciating the relief afforded by respite, when they can have 'time out' knowing their relative is being looked after (n=18)
- peace of mind when staff were well trained and delivered appropriate, person-centred care (n=15).

The above suggests that individually tailored services are required, as they are in urban areas. However, problems of distance, staff recruitment and few service options available compound the challenges of making high quality services available.

Innovations adopted to increase the availability of services

Three-quarters (76%) of service providers commented on innovative measures they had adopted to increase the availability of services to people with dementia and their carers.

The principal way in which availability of services had been increased was with the establishment of new services within the community (43%). Such services included the introduction of a telephone contact service, providing more beds or houses, new buildings, providing local day care and the introduction of a talking newspaper.

Providing information/education and engaging in awareness-raising activity was mentioned by 18 per cent of respondents as a way of increasing the availability of their service. Joint working was mentioned by 23 per cent of service providers as a way to increase the availability of services. However, the joint working methods mentioned both within the ways of working with other organisations, and as an innovative way to increase availability, did not demonstrate whether services have increased in availability and whether services have actually improved.

Successful innovations were attributed to a number of factors, including partnership working, improved working conditions for staff and managing personnel issues as innovations were being implemented. An observation from telephone interviews with service providers suggests that interpersonal issues are central to this process: 'It was implemented through good communication, presentations, face to face work.'

Accessibility of services

Problems in accessing services

The greatest difficulty service providers believed older people had in accessing services was distance between the user's home and the service location with just under half (43%) believing this to be a problem. Other areas of difficulty included lack of choice in services available (30%), shortage of appropriate skilled staff (23%) and the user having to meet the cost of the service (20%). Only a small amount of respondents indicated that there was a problem with a shortage of staff who speak community languages (9%) and a shortage of translated information (5%). However, since only a small percentage of the Scottish population are classified as minority communities (1.25%) (Scottish Executive 2001), this issue is likely to be significant for those members of the population whose first or chosen language is not English. Figures for older people whose chosen language is Gaelic do not appear to be available. However, there are 86,000 Gaelic speakers in Scotland for whom a lack of translated information and staff speaking their language could be a problem.[2]

Service providers perceived similar issues as problematic for older people with dementia, with similar numbers citing problems with distance (42%) and the cost of the service for the user (17%), although slightly more people believed there was a shortage of skilled staff (30%) and a lack of choices in services (36%) for older people with dementia compared to older people in general. Comments from telephone interviews illustrate problems with distance and skill deficits in relation to caring for people with dementia:

> Distance is a problem for the advocacy support. If for example there was one advocacy case, that can be one day's work.

> In relation to caring for demented patients, work needs to be done with unqualified carers to explore care issues involved in looking after clients with dementia, and attitudes and misunderstandings need to be addressed.

> There is a shortage of staff which causes ongoing problems. This is perhaps a national issue rather than a local one, but the fact that the council operates in a rural area may add to the problem.

> All links with choice. It's a rural community and people don't have a choice of five or six different services.

This highlights specific difficulties in providing a service in remote and rural Scotland as well as problems in providing high quality dementia care provision (see Table 2.4).

Table 2.4 Access difficulties		
Access difficulties	*N*	*%*
Distance between user's home and service location	36	29
Lack of choice in services available	31	25
Shortage of appropriate skilled staff	26	21
Cost of service to be met by service user	15	12
Shortage of staff who speak community languages	7	6
Shortage of translated information	4	4
Lack of specialist provision for people with dementia	2	2
Inequality of service	1	1
Shortage of funding	1	1
Transport availability/arrangements	1	1
TOTAL*	124	100

*Participants mentioned more than one difficulty, therefore the table adds up to more than the sum of the participants, or 100%.

Likewise all, bar five, carers mentioned some drawbacks to their current service provision. These included problems with staff (n=12), including staff shortages, inexperienced staff or poor interpersonal relationships; inappropriate provision which is not responsive to individual needs (n=11); feeling guilty about using respite (n=8); difficulties with co-ordination and communication (n=8); lack of information (n=8); service provision adding to rather than removing caring duties (n=6); and difficulties with transport to day care (n=3). Again, it highlights some of the problems in trying to provide person-centred care in a resource-constrained environment (Hill 2001).

During interviews with carers and PWD it was reported that not all PWD wished to use the services offered to them. Some participants (n=3) did not attend day care when offered as they either found it too tiring or were not attracted to group activities. One participant did not want to use temporary respite again as she had not enjoyed it. Three participants rejected the idea of personal care, as they did not like the idea of having their personal space invaded, and two participants did not want home help, again arguing they were able to fend for themselves. In the words of one participant: 'But she doesn't want a home help, she likes having things to do on a rainy day' (field-noted interview).

Carers also rejected some services. Most frequently mentioned was refusing offers of temporary residential respite (n=13) which they felt was too distressing for their relatives to use. This can be linked to the lack of appropriate care as illustrated by this quote: 'The only way they seem to be able to handle somebody in [wife's] situation is to put her into a psychiatric unit and lock her in a cell and I wasn't going to ask for it if that was what was going to happen' (taped interview with carer). Other services that were rejected include offers of day care respite (n=12), long-term residential care (n=5), personal care or home help (n=5) and medication (n=3).

The majority of carers felt they knew where to go for assistance if they needed it. Interestingly, they tended to highlight personal networks and their GP as access points for further services rather than state or voluntary service providers specific to dementia. This becomes understandable as six participants rejected the label of 'dementia', although all of the sample have been formally diagnosed with the condition. Access to services was a particular issue for one participant who struggled to get a diagnosis of their condition, which in turn had considerable impact on their access to services.

People with dementia and carers also discussed how access to services was connected with receiving a diagnosis of dementia. In total, ten carers and one PWD discussed how they struggled to get a diagnosis for the condition. This meant that, without a diagnosis, they were not able to access support mechanisms and services. Notably, many of these carers lobbied for medical attention and services as they had been able to identify the condition through previous experience caring for other family members or friends. In total, five carers sought services themselves, rather than being referred through medical or social work channels.

Gaps in services provided

The majority of service providers (72%) identified gaps in service provision with less than one-fifth (19%) indicating that service coverage is adequate. Gaps identified by service providers were mainly in their own service provision but six respondents indicated that there were gaps in services they perceived to be the responsibility of other service providers. Frequently reported gaps in services mentioned by service providers were:

- not enough services for people living at home, including day care provision (39%)
- lack of specialist services for people with dementia (27%)
- lack of long stay care provision, including residential, nursing home and hospital beds (26%)
- a lack of specialist training and recruitment and retention of suitable staff (10%)
- concern that existing services did not meet existing needs of service users (8%)
- lack of transport for service users (5%).

Equally illuminating were the gaps in services identified by people with dementia. Fifty per cent of people with dementia named gaps in provision, with half of these participants wanting more or different activities at their day centres or more days at the centre, two wanting to ensure access to their particular doctor, one wanting more attention at day care and one wanting more appropriate housing. However, careful inspection of the interview transcripts indicates additional 'gaps' not directly articulated. Thus, a lack of transport was an issue for five participants; three participants wanted services that would allow them to bring their pets; two wanted more day trips out; another two wanted help with vision impairment; one wanted help with their garden; and one needed modifications to their bathroom.

Likewise, 78 per cent of carers identified gaps in the PWD service provision. The most common issues raised were: need for more respite time (n=12); problems with transport to day care (n=10); need for more appropriate respite, including overnight respite in the home (n=9); lack of information about disease (n=6); lack of support for carer, particularly in the early stages of the disease (n=6); medical staff without specific expertise in dementia (n=5); lack of trained local staff (n=5); no carers support group (n=3); lack of financial support for carers, particularly those who give up their jobs (n=2); and a lack of local long-term residential care (n=2).

Accessing services poses unique challenges to rural areas due to the time it can take to get to a service, the need for transport to use a service and the need for local services which may encompass a wide service provider geographical area. Many of the gaps identified in services are no doubt common to urban areas; however, transport in particular is a gap that emerges when the service on offer may be a three-hour round trip away.

Opportunities and problems providing services in remote and rural areas

Service providers reported on innovations they had introduced to improve services as well as further opportunities and problems they felt rurality imposed on their provision.

Innovations by service providers to improve services

Transport was a key innovation for 30 per cent of service providers. Service providers had elected to use either one or a combination of local transport schemes (volunteer drivers, taxis, ambulances and staff members' own cars) to overcome difficulties for service users accessing services.

To make the service offered more accessible to those living in remote rural locations 26 per cent of service providers had developed outreach and/or locally based services. A further 14 per cent of respondents had developed and extended services delivered in the service user's own home. This was reinforced during four of the eleven telephone interviews. For example:

> If the clients need to travel a distance, the home carer has extra effort in getting the client ready; this along with the travel time to the facility and home again makes the client tired – some relatives say it is just not worth it. Home care in this instance is better for all concerned.

Service providers (14%) mentioned joint working as their innovation to improve accessibility of services. Joint working is an issue that cuts across the accessibility, availability and funding of services. Nine per cent of service providers had utilised technology to deliver their services, including the Internet and the telephone. A further 8 per cent had adapted premises and facilities to accommodate physically frail clients.

Opportunities

Forty-eight service providers (56%) commented on opportunities available to them when delivering services in rural areas. Forty per cent of service providers felt that joint working was more of a possibility in rural areas. This was due to a combination of the community networks available, the geographical location, local knowledge and shared working in areas such as transport.

Some service providers (14%) felt that there were increased opportunities for more effective service delivery if the respondent was the only service provider, engaged in outreach work, or was a well-known figure within the community since they did not have to negotiate with other providers. Fifteen per cent felt that locally provided services created opportunities for better knowledge of clients' needs. Eight per cent were however sceptical about any opportunities available in rural areas and the potential for creating more positive ways of delivering services in the future.

PWD and carers also argued that rural areas presented opportunities for excellent service provision. In particular, both carers (n=17) and participants with dementia (n=5) felt that living in rural areas meant that service provision was personalised and able to respond to individual conditions. Their comments reinforced the service providers' comments about overlapping personal and professional social networks – for example, 'Edward and his sister felt that the man from the Social Work Department would have a good knowledge of his community, and would know who needed what' (interview with PWD). Indeed, 13 participants explicitly argued that service provision in rural areas was better than in a city for this reason. Furthermore, many carers and PWD felt that rural living offered them a better quality of life, which made up for problems with service provision in rural areas.

Problems

Seventy-eight per cent of respondents (67) described problems they face when delivering services in rural areas. Over half (52%) of the respondents stated that transport was a key problem arising from the geographical dispersion of the population and the travel distance between the service user's home and place of service delivery. In addition the costs of travelling (for both users and providers) were seen as problematic. Lack of funding was a frequently cited problem (36%), encompassing shortage of funding and lack of adequate resources. Staffing issues, namely recruitment and retention of appropriate staff, were cited as a problem for 28 per cent of respondents, with shortages of volunteers specified by a further nine per cent of respondents. Another problem was a lack of places or appropriate facilities (12%). Comments from telephone interviews with service providers highlight distance and cost problems that can be inherent when providing rural services:

'Transport is costly. These costs need to be taken into account when providing a service. This is not the same in the city centre.'

Time was also highlighted in the questionnaires with some clients' journeys reported to take up to three hours: 'A trip can take half an hour to 40 minutes. Sometimes need to balance, take one person on a long distance or four close together.'

Carers and PWD also felt that the major disadvantages raised above, such as transport problems, staffing shortages, lack of choice and lack of specialist care, are made worse by the issue of distances between the client and the place of service delivery. Low population density has implications for recruiting staff and for resource allocations, again explaining some of the drawbacks of current provision and the service gaps expressed by our participants. While we found evidence of significant informal support from family and friends, only three carers mentioned support by community organisations (local church and Rotary Club) and even then this support was limited. This finding makes our understanding of rural support networks more ambiguous, indicating informal support is more individualised and contingent than an ideology of a caring community might suggest.

Conclusions

This chapter has gone some way to identify key issues as experienced across a broad spectrum of services. Health and social policy in Scotland needs to consider a rural dimension to training and education, as well as specific dementia training, to ensure practitioners in remote and rural areas are appropriately skilled. Recruitment and retention of skilled staff in remote and rural areas is crucial for the development and delivery of quality services for PWD and their carers in the future. The lack of available services and difficulties in accessing services need to be examined against demographic profiles and the effects that lack of choice or access can have on the health status of older people, people with dementia and their carers.

The findings from this work highlight two aspects for future research with service users in remote and rural areas. First, that it is possible to give voice to this particular marginalised group. The findings briefly outlined above indicate that people with dementia and their carers in remote and rural Scotland are both willing and able to articulate their needs as a user group. Second, the importance of service provision to be flexible and person centred (Kitwood 1997) responds dynamically to the changing needs of the individual participants. Difficulties imposed by rurality (distance, geographical dispersal of client group, staff retention and recruitment) should not obscure these two points. Service providers, carers and PWD were all aware of the need for flexible and appropriate service provision.

We have indicated the importance of this field of study, which has increasing policy and political relevance in our ageing society in Scotland. We have demonstrated that it is possible to set out on the journey but conclude we still have a long way to go.

Acknowledgements

The research reported on here was sponsored by the Carnegie Trust for the Universities of Scotland, Royal Society of Edinburgh/Lloyds TSB Foundation and University of Stirling Faculty Development Fund.

We wish to acknowledge the input of a large collaborative team, particularly Sylvia Cox, Anne Mason and Annetta Smith, in the conduct of the research referred to above.

Notes

1   Aberdeenshire Council (2000) *Community Care – Central Locality Plan.* www.aberdeenshire.gov.uk/ communitycare/central/part7_2.htm.

2   www.geo.ed.ac.uk/home/scotland/gaelic.html.

References

Aberdeenshire Council (2000) *Community Care – Central Locality Plan.* www.aberdeenshire.gov.uk/communitycare/central/part7_2.htm.

Armstrong, G.E. (2002) *Adding Life to Years.* Edinburgh: Scottish Executive.

Camicioli, R., Willert, P., Lear, J., Grossman, S., Kaye, J. and Butterfield, P. (2000) 'Dementia in rural primary care practices in Lake County, Oregon.' *Journal of Geriatric Psychiatry and Neurology 13,* 87–92.

Cook, A. (2002) 'Using video observation to include the experiences of people with dementia in research.' In H. Wilkinson (ed) *The Perspectives of People with Dementia: Research Methods and Motivations.* London: Jessica Kingsley Publishers.

Corner, L. (2002) 'Including people with dementia: advisory networks and user panels.' In H. Wilkinson (ed) *The Perspectives of People with Dementia: Research Methods and Motivations.* London: Jessica Kingsley Publishers.

Dementia Services Development Centre (1998) *Supporting People with Dementia and their Carers in Rural Communities.* Conference proceedings. Stirling: University of Stirling.

Gilmour, H. (2002) 'Dementia in a social context.' *Journal of Dementia Care,* Jan/Feb, 10.

Gilmour, H., Gibson, F. and Campbell, J. (2003) 'People with dementia in a rural community: issues of prevalence and community care policy.' *Dementia 2*, 2, 245–263.

Glendinning, A., Nuttal, M., Hendry, L., Kloep, M. and Wood, S. (2003) 'Rural communities and well being: a good place to grow up?' *The Sociological Review 51*, 1, 129–156.

Goldsmith, M. (1996) *Hearing the Voice of People with Dementia: Opportunities and Obstacles.* London: Jessica Kingsley Publishers.

Hill, H. (2001) 'Why is it so hard to focus on the person? Issues involved in implementing person centred care.' *Signpost 5*, 3, 16–18.

Hope, S., Anderson, S. and Sawyer, B. (2000) *The Quality of Services in Rural Scotland.* Scottish Executive Central Research Unit. Edinburgh: The Stationery Office.

Innes, A. and Capstick, A. (2001) 'Communication and personhood.' In C. Cantley (ed) *Handbook of Dementia Care.* Buckingham: Open University Press.

Innes, A., Cox, S., Mason, A. and Smith, A. (2002) *Service Provision for People with Dementia in Remote and Rural Scotland.* Stirling: University of Stirling.

Kitwood, T. (1997) *Dementia Reconsidered: The Person Comes First.* Buckingham: Open University Press.

Le Mesurier, N. and Duncan, G. (2000) 'Over the hills and far away: providing accessible day care services for older people in rural areas.' *Managing Community Care 8*, 4, 33–37.

Nolan, M., Ryan, T., Enderby, P. and Reid, D. (2002) 'Towards a more inclusive vision of dementia care practice and research.' *Dementia 1*, 2, 193–211.

O'Reilly, M.T. and Strong, J. (1997) 'Caring for someone with dementia in a rural town. Part 2: Services.' *Australian Journal on Ageing 16*, 4, 194–197.

Paul, L., Johnson, A.O. and Cranston, G.M. (2000) 'A successful video conference satellite program: providing nutritional information on dementia to rural caregivers.' *Educational Gerontology 26*, 415–425.

Proctor, G. (2001) 'Listening to older women with dementia.' *Disability and Society 16*, 3, 361–376.

Scottish Executive (2001) *Scottish Household Survey.* Edinburgh: Scottish Executive National Statistics.

Shucksmith, M. and Murphy, C. (eds) (1999) *Rural Audit: A Health Check on Rural Britain.* Commissioned by The Rural Group of Labour MPs, Arkleton Centre for Rural Development Research, Aberdeen.

Sjobeck, B. and Isacsson, A. (1994) 'Caring for demented elderly in rural primary health care.' *Scandinavian Journal of Caring Sciences 8*, 1, 29–37.

Wenger, G.C. (2001) 'Myths and realities of ageing in rural Britain.' *Ageing and Society 21*, 117–130.

West Highland Project (1992) *Living with Disability in Remote Areas: A Survey of the Support Required by Some Rural Families with Special Needs.* Glasgow: Scottish Society for the Mentally Handicapped.

Wilkinson, H. (ed) (2002) *The Perspectives of People with Dementia: Research Methods and Motivations.* London: Jessica Kingsley Publishers.

CHAPTER 3

Improving Domiciliary Care for People with Dementia and their Carers: The Raising the Standard Project

Noni Cobban

Background

Government policy has been shifting the emphasis of care services away from institutional settings and towards home-based services (Department of Health 1998; Scottish Office 1999). Home care services can expect the number of people with dementia to grow over the coming years in line with growth in our ageing population (Alzheimer's Society 1997; Moriarty and Webb 2000). In response to these demographic trends and policy shifts, home care organisations are facing new challenges to provide a wider range of more flexible services (Accounts Commission for Scotland 2001). The traditional 'home help' services which provided domestic and household assistance are now increasingly providing complex and intimate personal care packages and targeting these newer services towards those with the greatest need (Clark, Dyer and Horwood 1998; Godfrey *et al.* 2000; Department of Health 2002). Home care staff now face greater responsibilities in their day-to-day work, which at times can be more akin to nursing than to domestic help (Accounts Commission for Scotland 2001; Taylor 2001). In addition, the home care industry will be formally regulated by the regulating bodies for care services, with employers under pressure for their staff to achieve at least minimum levels of vocational qualifications in care (Department of Health 2003;

TOPSS England 2000). Despite these moves, there has been scant regard paid to the specific training or support needs of home care staff in working with people with dementia (Moriarty and Webb 2000).

Home care has historically had a low status in the hierarchy of social services departments. This, however, is changing as home care services develop to meet the needs of increasingly vulnerable people. People with dementia, with complex care needs, are now able to live longer in the community, and it is necessary to find ways and means of helping home care organisations and their frontline workers to develop the appropriate knowledge, skills and attitudes to support this client group.

This chapter will outline the main issues in home care generally; for home care staff; and in delivering home care to people with dementia. We then describe the aims and methodology of our study in this field – the Raising the Standard Project. This chapter concludes with a summary of our main findings and the three core recommendations arising from the study.

What is home care?

There is a general consensus that most people prefer to live in their own home where they have control over how they manage the most private and intimate aspects of their lives. The home and social environment are key factors, unique to home care, which influence a person's potential to maintain independence and autonomy over their activities of daily living. People who need help to look after themselves or their home may have to turn to providers of home care for this help. In doing so, they should feel confident that anyone whom they allow into their home is reliable, trustworthy and competent to do what they want them to do. Service users report that being treated with respect, courtesy and maintaining confidentiality are quality indicators: 'It was clear...that relationships formed between service users and home care workers play a major part in the success of the home care service' (Accounts Commission for Scotland 2001, p.25).

Home care services are provided by all sectors, local authorities, private and voluntary providers. They are diverse and wide ranging from provision of domestic and practical support around the house to complex, personal and nursing care tasks. There is evidence that workers are increasingly being asked to undertake healthcare tasks such as assisting with catheters, medication and specialist feeding (Taylor 2001). The common factor in all these tasks is that they are things which people would normally prefer to do for themselves but cannot manage without some help. Significant changes have taken place in home care since the implementation of community care reforms in the early 1990s. The pace, scale and scope of these changes have varied across the UK and there is considerable variation between local authorities. In England, the shift from local authority provision to contracting with the independent sector has resulted in more than 51 per cent of home care services being purchased from external providers (Nuffield Institute for Health and PSSRU 2001), compared with 72 per cent provision by local authorities in Scotland (Scottish Executive 2002). There has been an increasing trend towards targeting service users with high dependency needs and prioritising personal care tasks at the expense of practical support with housework (Godfrey *et al.* 2000). The result of this targeting has been an increase in the number of people receiving more intensive home care packages with an overall reduction in the number of people who receive a home care service. This is despite successive household surveys which show that it is the domestic tasks that cause people more difficulty than self-care, and that these problems are exacerbated with increasing age (Godfrey *et al.* 2000). Another trend which has grown with the development of the market economy for purchasing care has been local authority reliance on spot contracting of 'time slots' to provide a particular task. This style of contracting conflicts with the aspirations of policy makers to offer user choice over how and when their care is provided and the development of person-centred care packages.

For most of us the meaning of home is symbolic of our privacy and independence. It is a 'special space', and how we order our lives therein is linked to our sense of identity, security and our status. Julia Twigg gives a sensitive and fascinating insight into the taboos of personal care – looking after our own bodies – and examines what actually happens when the professional, formal world of the care sector enters this intensely private, bodily based domain of 'getting up, dressing, eating, sleeping, excreting' (Twigg 2000). Home care touches on the most private and often intimate aspects of people's lives. The manner in which help is offered and provided, the perception of each person's feelings and the dynamic relationship that is created between the giver and receiver of help are of at least equal significance (Fox 1999; Greenwood, Loewenthal and Rose 2001; Walmsley 1998).

Who are the home care workers?

The world of home care lies between the aspirations of policy makers 'as the cornerstone of community care' and the low status it is given by many professional staff. Home care workers are the basis on which the desired shift in balance to non-institutional care will depend and yet, despite this, they remain under-trained, under-managed, under-paid and under-valued. The home care workforce is unique in that staff, mainly without qualifications, carry out their day-to-day activities out of sight of any line management or supervision. The job requires staff to be patient, resourceful, flexible and willing to undertake a range of tasks from house cleaning to intimate personal care. Ebenstein (1998), who interviewed home care workers to seek their views of what makes the 'best' home care worker, found that the qualities most highly rated were patience, respect and compassion. They also identified self-awareness with the ability to reflect and understand that they should not take things personally. This study found that the sources of job satisfaction stem from seeing an improvement in the lives of the service users and enjoying close relationships with them.

Most home care workers are female and many work part-time (UNISON 2003). Estimates suggest there are between 200,000 and 300,000 home care workers in the UK (TOPSS England 2000), and it is an ageing workforce with 94 per cent over the age of 35 and almost one-third are over 55 (Taylor 2001; UNISON 2003). The work of home care has been stereotyped as unskilled work that anyone can do, and is accordingly low paid (Henwood 2001; UNISON 2003). Yet the recent predominance of personal care over domestic chores has meant that home care is now a physically and mentally demanding job (Bell 2001). The UNISON home care worker survey (Taylor 2001) found that 67 per cent report that their work is predominantly personal care against 16 per cent reporting this five years ago; 75 per cent report that they work with people with dementia and that they are increasingly undertaking health-related activities such as catheter care, medications, dressings and stoma care. Workers are frequently dealing with stressful or emotionally demanding situations (Arts *et al.* 2001), often under constant time pressure to complete tasks during a visit with higher levels of individual responsibility. They have to think on their feet, often being faced with making decisions by themselves (Trojan and Yonge 1993).

Home care for people with dementia

The dual aims of reducing institutionalisation (Nolan, Ingram and Watson 2002) and moving towards a positive person-centred approach to enhance the quality and meaning of life for the person with dementia and their carer (Lightbody and Gilhooly 1997) has resulted in an expectation that generic home care services will be able to move away from a pessimistic, least risk approach to care provision for this group. Kitwood (1997) lists the five important needs of people with dementia as inclusion, attachment, comfort, identity and occupation. Good dementia care is grounded in the ability of care workers to maintain effective communication with individuals as one human being to another (Allan 2000). Evidence from service users with dementia also suggests that how a home care worker carries out a task is as important to them as the activity itself. They value the relationships with the home care worker as much as the practical help given (Ebenstein 1998; Moriarty and Webb 2000). The interpersonal skills of home care workers are crucial to the success of a home care intervention (Accounts Commission for Scotland 2001) and are key to the success of home care services for people with dementia (Herbert 1997; Olsson and Hallberg 1998). This is not least because the attitudes, actions and reactions of staff can have a significant effect on so-called symptoms of dementia (Kitwood 1997). Olsson and Hallberg (1998) studied the role of supervision of home care workers engaged in work with people with dementia and found that the relationship between staff and the person with dementia stood out as central to the quality of care. This relationship was enhanced by supervision, which increased the workers' reflective and analytical capacity, their knowledge about dementia and improved their collaboration with others.

Other factors identified as affecting workers in this field were lack of co-operation between home care and other professionals and the lack of resources and time to fulfil their role. The tendency for home care to be commissioned on the basis of task-focused 'time slots' (Godfrey *et al.* 2000) can impede the process of developing communication and relationships. This makes it difficult for home care workers to address the less tangible, relational aspects of care (Allan 2001).

Lack of time is a commonly reported problem by care workers involved in dementia care (Goldsmith 1996; Olsson and Hallberg 1998) and it has been suggested that, in some circumstances, lack of time can be a convenient excuse for staff who appear to feel safer if not involved in the feelings and needs of people with dementia (Goldsmith 1996). Relating effectively to people with dementia can pose particular problems for staff who have been taught to keep a 'professional distance' (Loveday 1998). Such staff are likely to require a high degree of support, to lower their own defensive barriers and reflect on their own personal responses. This requires a high level of skill on the part of the supervisor (Packer 2001). Arguably, if staff learn about the physiology of dementia and the neurological impairment involved, it could help to put supposedly bizarre behaviours into context (Aveyard 2001). Such knowledge could help staff to realise that hurtful comments or odd behaviours are not directed at them but are a consequence of impairment in the brain. This could aid them in approaching such problems positively through interpreting behaviour as a form of communication. For those workers who, over a period of time, develop a knowledge and awareness of their clients with dementia as real people, it is a job with personal rewards. Foremost among these is the satisfaction derived from enjoying this close relationship and witnessing improvements in their lives as a result of the care provided (Ebenstein 1998).

Bamford and Bruce (2000), in consulting people with dementia about their views of home care, found that along with the relationship developed with their home care worker, it was important to them to maintain a strong sense of being in control. While remaining at home was an important symbol of control in itself, service users with dementia wanted to have a greater say in how their home care service was delivered. They wanted help to maximise their autonomy and to be treated normally as an individual, with value and respect. Their sense of personal identity was strongly bound up with their ability to fulfil traditional roles such as cooking and cleaning, and home care was accepted reluctantly, leaving some people with dementia feeling 'redundant' or undermining their sense of autonomy. They favoured a 'low key' approach to their home care, where they were not made to feel that someone was doing them a favour.

The role and views of family carers are another aspect of caring for people with dementia at home in which home care workers have to balance the needs, wishes and rights of people with dementia with those of any family carers. Some family carers may be reluctant to accept services until they reach the point at which they have begun to experience high degrees of stress or poor psychological health (Webb, Moriarty and Levin 1998). Therefore home care workers may find they have to deal sensitively with a carer who may be feeling upset, stressed or guilty for allowing services to become involved. There is always a danger of undermining the carer's role by appearing to 'take over', or diminishing their sense of success or expertise (Nolan *et al.* 2002). Conflicts of interest between a carer's wishes and those of the person with dementia can need careful negotiation by home care workers.

Raising the Standard action research project

Raising the Standard was an action research project that took place between August 2000 and October 2002 looking at ways to improve home care for people with dementia and their carers.

The aims of this project were as follows:

- to understand the issues and problems facing generic home care organisations and staff in relation to caring for people with dementia
- to review current UK developments in home care
- to make proposals on a model, which could make a positive difference to the home care received by people with dementia and their carers
- to develop materials or methods to assist with the implementation of this model.

This qualitative study comprised three stages. The first stage was a review of the research literature, policy documents and existing training materials. This helped us to understand the political and policy context in which home care organisations are operating. The review also led us to question the extent to which home care staff working in mainstream home care organisations with people with dementia were adequately prepared to provide person-centred care. We recognised that much was written about home care at an organisational or higher level, but care workers were a group whose perspectives were under-represented in research and policy (Jacques and Innes 1998; Moriarty and Webb 2000). Hence we were keen to listen to the experiences and issues as described by those staff directly involved in the delivery of care.

The second stage of the research employed a variety of methods to try to uncover the key issues and themes in delivering home care to people with dementia. Initially we publicised the project by circulating an information leaflet to home care providers and trainers in the United Kingdom. We requested contact details from those interested in taking part in the study and used the returns to develop a database. We selected seven sites, from the database, to carry out focus group interviews to seek views about dementia care from staff working in the field. These sites were in both urban and rural settings and from local authority and independent sector providers. Three of the focus groups were with home care workers only, two with the frontline managers and two were mixed groups with both home care workers and their frontline managers. There was an average of 12 participants in each group.

Information from the focus groups was supplemented in a number of ways: telephone interviews were held with two home care managers and three trainers from the independent and public sectors; face-to-face interviews with dementia care co-ordinators working with a local healthcare co-operative in

Scotland; and attendance as an observer at one-day training courses for home care workers, to gain an insight into the training experience of home care staff.

We were also interested in contrasting the home care workers' experience with a group of staff in another sector with a similar profile. Although a strictly like for like comparison with another industry was not possible, the retail sector staff profile is thought to be similar to that of home care staff in terms of age, gender and the part-time nature of the work. Furthermore, as supermarkets are widely believed to compete with social care employers for recruitment, we considered that there would be sufficient, relevant common factors. We interviewed a human resources manager from a national supermarket chain and held a group interview with 12 shop floor staff in a supermarket in Central Scotland.

The data gathered from these various interviews and observations in stage two were used as the basis for developing questionnaires for the postal survey which formed stage three of the research. This survey was designed to gain a more detailed understanding from home care workers, frontline managers and trainers about their own perspectives of their job, and about the support and training which frontline workers received in relation to working with people with dementia. The questionnaires were piloted with each of these groups and comments from the returns were reflected in the final version. This was distributed to 400 home care workers, 200 frontline managers and 44 trainers in all four countries of the UK. The overall response rate was 12 per cent, with home care workers returning 12 per cent, frontline managers 11 per cent and trainers 16 per cent.

What we found

The majority of mainstream home care staff who participated in our project provided care for people with a known form of dementia. Staff also reported visiting other people at home with some level of confusion but without a formal diagnosis of dementia. The views of the respondents can be summarised into four main themes: difficulties experienced in doing the job, support and supervision, training and finally issues relating to working with people with dementia.

Difficulties experienced doing the job

Home care workers believe that they have low status in the workplace: 'We are labelled as cleaners and shoppers. It's the bottom of the pile' and 'Pay's dreadful. They need to reward you. It's nursing on the cheap. Dressings and drops...'

Although they feel undervalued by their employers, they believe they are highly valued by the service users. They report high levels of job satisfaction derived from their relationships with service users and the feeling that they are helping people in need.

A significant theme, which arose during the group interviews in stage two, was the constant pressure of time the workers are under and the task approach to arranging services, which affects their ability to provide person-centred care. This was also reflected in the responses to the questionnaires in stage three. Staff were concerned that the time they can spend with a person has an impact on the person's independence: 'We are robbing them of the skills they have because of the time.'

Staff described working in a culture of inflexible policies such as not being allowed to change a client's light bulbs or clean their curtains; unclear levels of responsibility for assisting with medication; working with faulty cleaning equipment; and providing cover for staff who are absent. We were aware that many workers felt a high degree of responsibility towards the people they visited, even outwith work hours. A few home care workers reported having given out their personal phone numbers to clients or family carers.

Home care workers often sought guidance in practical care matters. Several workers spoke highly of receiving 'hands on' training from Marie Curie nurses or district nurses who had helped them find ways to overcome particular difficulties or provided skills instruction. When questioned about whether they could see a similar type of support for people with dementia, workers expressed a desire for appropriate help or support at the actual time they were experiencing a difficulty.

Support and supervision

Supervision and support of this staff group, who are largely unqualified and are working alone with vulnerable people, should be an important factor in the management of a home care service. However, planned supervision sessions frequently give way to the higher priority of meeting the organisational demands of the service. Staff are rarely accompanied while carrying out their work to appraise their performance or identify skills gaps. Frontline managers are dependent on staff reporting problems back to them at the office base. Despite these difficulties home care workers report that when they need to contact their manager for support it is forthcoming in most cases.

For home care workers time to come together with peers or supervisors to talk about their work is very rare yet very welcome when it occurs. This was particularly apparent during the informal contact at the end of the group interviews when home care workers were meeting each other face to face for the first time. This isolation from colleagues is a problem unique to this dispersed workforce.

The lack of formal supervision and appraisal in the work of home care organisations contrasts sharply with the impression we gained from the group interview with the staff in a large national supermarket. This group of staff conveyed the sense that they were well supported with a clear understanding of their status and opportunities with the company. All members of staff received regular supervision and had individual training plans. The group we interviewed were well motivated, felt they were valued by the organisation but, again in contrast to home care workers, they felt undervalued by their customers.

Training

The size of this workforce and the low qualification base presents home care organisations with a considerable challenge for addressing the training and development needs of their staff. Managers reported having difficulty in releasing staff for training and saw their main priority as ensuring that mandatory training took place. All staff reported that they had received training in moving and handling, health and safety, food hygiene and first aid.

The shift towards supporting more vulnerable people with increasing personal care needs will need new skill levels from staff but this has not been accompanied by adequate resources in terms of money and accessibility of training opportunities for staff. Some organisations have made some progress with achieving generic national vocational qualifications with their staff but, overall, numbers remain small. For example, an organisation employing 1200 home care workers has achieved qualifications for 250 staff which means that nearly 80 per cent remain unqualified. Staff and line managers also reported that, where the role of workplace assessment is combined with other home care management and co-ordinating duties, the day-to-day pressures of the service take priority over planned assessment and supervision sessions. This means that it can take up to two years for a candidate to complete their portfolio of evidence for a qualification. In organisations where qualification targets are a priority, resources are consequently concentrated on the staff working towards the qualification at the expense of the majority. Staff reported that they had difficulty getting on training courses and that it was their perception that older workers were disadvantaged.

In terms of training resources, we found that there is information about training and learning for the care sector; there are training resources for dementia care – albeit with the focus mainly directed towards staff working in residential settings; and there is now an emphasis on training and developing an award framework for home care. However, the links between training, dementia and home care are missing. Despite the number of dementia care training materials and courses available, many staff said they were either not aware of these or had difficulty knowing how to access them. For those home care workers who had received training in dementia, it was mainly a 'one-off' course lasting from a half day to three days. Where short training courses like this had taken place, staff reported positive changes to their work, although the effects of the training appeared to diminish over time unless refresher courses were available: 'It was something to do with principles and respect. It was four years ago. I can't remember.'

Working with people with dementia

I would just like to note that when I first started working with clients who suffered from dementia I felt very unhappy and out of my depth, feeling quite helpless sometimes, as I was very often unable to understand their needs but during the past 13 years I have worked with many clients with this awful disease and have gained great knowledge and self-satisfaction. (Quote from a home care worker)

It was notable that information from the interviews and questionnaires (stages two and three) showed that home care workers felt they had learnt most about dementia from the people they cared for, or from experiential learning on the job. Several such comments were:

- 'hands on has given me the most experience'
- 'by facing it every day and realising that everyone's dementia is different'
- 'training was beneficial but working and gaining experience with dementia clients has taught me how to cope with clients in a realistic manner'
- 'I went out with another worker and I learnt more than going on a course'

- 'we need more hands-on training than having to go home and write it up'.

For many workers, getting to know the person and personality behind the dementia label over a period of time was considered to be the most important factor that helped them provide person-centred care. Some home care workers expressed good understanding regarding the needs of individual service users, speaking of them as individuals with capacities, needs and wishes. Many spoke warmly of the relationships they had developed over time with clients who had dementia and of the reciprocal benefits of investing time and energy in this during their visits.

The views and assumptions of some others regarding the nature of dementia were clearly constructed through a lens of seeing older people with dementia in terms of their deficits, and to be compared with the 'norm' of a healthy younger adult. Such negative conceptions would be likely to result in subtle forms of disempowerment for the person with dementia, albeit unin-tentionally. Staff were generally aware of the negative consequences for clients of a time-based service led approach in terms of enforcing their dependence. They reported that lack of time created difficulties when unexpected problems cropped up. A number of home care workers said they went beyond the contracted tasks and visited clients with dementia in their own free time to make sure they were all right.

When caring for people with dementia, they also reported that they are faced with common day-to-day problems such as difficulty in gaining access to the home or in acceptance by the person that they need help with either personal care or domestic support. They expressed anxiety about accusations of theft from clients' homes which underlines the vulnerability and isolation of this type of work. Frontline managers referred to concerns about difficult and aggressive behaviour although this was not an issue that arose from the home care workers themselves.

What could be done to improve domiciliary care for people with dementia and their carers?

It was evident from our research that home care workers are under-trained, under-managed, and under-valued for the work that they do supporting people with dementia. Additionally the low qualification base, the dispersed nature of this workforce and a lack of resources to accomplish much more than the mandatory training made it clear that there would be no simple solution to training and development of home care staff to work with people with dementia. The issues involved for large generic home care services in providing person-centred care are complex and varied, and the interventions required to engender appropriate knowledge, skills and attitudes in frontline staff run deeper than the straightforward provision of training (Lintern, Woods and Phair 2000). The following recommendations aim to take account of the need to find ways in which an awareness and understanding of people with dementia could be conveyed to and sustained in all staff working in home care in a way which would influence the culture of home care with regard to people with dementia.

Recommendation 1: The perspective of people with dementia should be incorporated into induction and basic training undertaken by all new home care workers

We know that the main training emphasis is on the mandatory areas of induction, health and safety, food hygiene, and moving and handling. We concluded that incorporating a basic awareness of dementia into this induction training would start a culture which is empathetic to the needs of this group of people and would assist staff to understand how to balance safety with maintaining independence. Staff should be helped to consider the effect of using equipment for moving and handling on a person who has difficulty in making sense of what is happening to them. This proposal is made in recognition of the importance for dementia care of creating an environment which educates staff in the importance of attitudes and relationships (Greenwood *et al.* 2001), and doing so early on in their career. Such training is necessary to provide a framework for any knowledge or skills training received at a later date if person-centred care is to be a reality (Aveyard 2001).

Recommendation 2: Field supervisors, whose job is separate from day-to-day service organisation demands, should carry out ongoing supervision and development of frontline staff

In addition to basic training, staff were saying that they need support and skills instruction on an ongoing basis. They need immediate 'on the job' instruction to address any skill gaps if the condition of the person they are caring for deteriorates or they are assigned to a new person whose needs require new skills from the member of staff. It is also essential that training and education in dementia care is supported and followed up. We suggest the introduction of a field supervisor, a role which is separate from day-to-day organisation, to provide ongoing mentoring, skills instruction, supervision, support and assessment of practice. The critical skills required for this role will be advanced skills in personal care, a sound working knowledge of the needs of people with dementia, and good communication skills which motivate and value staff.

Recommendation 3: Locality-based dementia specialist workers should be made accessible to home care workers for ongoing skills training and advice

Home care workers told us that when they cared for people with a terminal illness they had the opportunity to learn new practical skills from working with Macmillan or Marie Curie nurses. Similar models of community support for people with dementia are available in some areas: for example, the Admiral nurses in London and the Midlands who are dementia specialists providing a similar function to that of Macmillan nurses, and the dementia care co-ordinators attached to local healthcare co-operatives in a Scottish health board. We are suggesting that locality-based dementia specialist workers should be available for advice, guidance and specialist skills instruction to home care workers on an individual basis. In addition, we think it makes sense that home care staff should have direct access to this support as needs arise, rather than the worker having to go through a range of intermediary and management staff. The success of this model would depend largely on the development of interprofessional relationships of mutual trust, respect and value for the skills that each could bring.

Conclusion

Home care for people with dementia is changing for the better (Moriarty and Webb 2000), but there is still much room for further improvement. Many of the new skills required in the field of dementia care appear not yet to have filtered down to frontline home care workers, perhaps not surprisingly as there has been little done by way of ensuring adequate resources in terms of money and accessibility of training, development and support for those staff.

Training packs and training courses have an important and valuable part to play in developing staff knowledge and understanding of dementia, but on their own they will not necessarily result in better care for people with dementia (Lintern *et al.* 2000). The links between training, support, supervision and individual personal development are critical to encourage staff in how they do their job and improve the valuable service they are providing to people with dementia who are living at home. This will be strongly affected by the way in which frontline staff are treated, inducted, managed, supported and advised (Herbert 1997; Kitwood 1997; Loveday 1998).

The recommendations we have made have drawn on evidence gathered from people working in the field. We believe they offer an approach that organisations could adopt, in whole or in part, as they endeavour to develop their services in ways that better reflect the needs of this client group and the needs of those staff most directly involved, while facilitating the empowerment of both.

References

Accounts Commission for Scotland (2001) *Homing in on Care: A Review of Home Care Services for Older People.* Edinburgh: Audit Scotland.

Allan, K. (2000) 'Drawing out views on services: a new staff-based approach.' *Journal of Dementia Care 8*, 6, 16–19.

Allan, K. (2001) *Communication and Consultation: Exploring Ways for Staff to Involve People with Dementia in Developing Services.* Bristol: The Policy Press and Joseph Rowntree Foundation.

Alzheimer's Society (1997) 'The prevalence of dementia.' *Alzheimer's Disease International Factsheet.* London: Alzheimer's Society.

Arts, S.E.J., Kerstra, A., van der Zee, J. and Abu-Saad, H.H. (2001) 'Quality of working life and workload in home help services.' *Nordic Journal of Caring Sciences 15*, 12–24.

Aveyard, B. (2001) 'Education and person-centred approaches to dementia care.' *Nursing Older People 12*, 10, 17–19.

Bamford, C. and Bruce, E. (2000) 'Defining the outcomes of community care: the perspectives of older people with dementia and their carers.' *Ageing and Society 20*, 534–570.

Bell, L. (2001) 'Competence in home care.' *Quality in Ageing 2*, 2, 13–20.

Clark, H., Dyer, S. and Horwood, J. (1998) *'That Bit of Help': The High Value of Low Level Preventative Services for Older People.* Bristol: The Policy Press in association with Community Care and Joseph Rowntree Foundation.

Department of Health (1998) *Modernising Social Services.* London: Department of Health.

Department of Health (2002) *Health and Personal Social Services Statistics: England* [available from www.doh.gov.uk/HPSSS/INDEX.HTM].

Department of Health (2003) *Domiciliary Care: National Standards and Regulations.* London: Department of Health.

Ebenstein, H. (1998) 'They were once like us: learning from home care workers who care for the elderly.' *Journal of Gerontological Social Work 30*, 3/4, 191–201.

Fox, N. (1999) *Beyond Health Postmodernism and Embodiment.* London: Free Association Press.

Godfrey, M., Randall, T., Long, A. and Grant, M. (2000) *Home Care: Review of Effectiveness and Outcomes.* University of Exeter: Centre for Evidence-Based Social Services.

Goldsmith, M. (1996) *Hearing the Voice of People with Dementia.* London: Jessica Kingsley Publishers.

Greenwood, D., Loewenthal, D. and Rose, T. (2001) 'A relational approach to providing care for a person suffering from dementia.' *Journal of Advanced Nursing 36*, 4, 583–590.

Henwood, M. (2001) *Future Imperfect? Report of the King's Fund Care and Support Inquiry.* London: King's Fund Publishing.

Herbert, G. (1997) 'Which hat should we wear today? Recruiting and developing the ideal workforce for dementia care.' In M. Marshall (ed) *State of the Art in Dementia Care.* London: Centre for Policy on Ageing.

Jacques, I. and Innes, A. (1998) 'Who cares about care assistant work?' *Journal of Dementia Care*, November/December, 33–37.

Kitwood, T. (1997) *Dementia Reconsidered: The Person Comes First.* Buckingham: Open University Press.

Lightbody, P. and Gilhooly, M. (1997) 'The continuing quest for predictions of breakdown of family care of elderly people with dementia.' In M. Marshall (ed) *State of the Art in Dementia Care.* London: Centre for Policy on Ageing.

Lintern, T., Woods, B. and Phair, L. (2000) 'Training is not enough to change care practice.' *Journal of Dementia Care 15*, March/April, 15–17.

Loveday, B. (1998) 'Training to promote person centred care.' *Journal of Dementia Care,*. March/April, 22–24.

Moriarty, J. and Webb, S. (2000) *Part of Their Lives: Community Care for Older People with Dementia.* Bristol: The Policy Press.

Nolan, M., Ingram, P. and Watson, R. (2002) 'Working with family carers of people with dementia.' *Dementia 1*, 1, 75–93.

Nuffield Institute for Health and PSSRU (2001) *Evidence Briefing Paper 6.* Leeds: Nuffield Institute for Health.

Olsson, A. and Hallberg, I.R. (1998) 'Caring for demented people in their homes or in sheltered accommodation as reflected on by home-care staff during clinical supervision sessions.' *Journal of Advanced Nursing 27*, 241–252.

Packer, T. (2001) 'Everyone wants something: recognising your own needs.' *Journal of Dementia Care*, January/February, 26–28.

Scottish Executive (2002) *Statistics Release: Home Care Services Scotland 2002.* Edinburgh: Scottish Executive.

Scottish Office (1999) *Aiming for Excellence: Modernising Social Work Services in Scotland.* Edinburgh: The Stationery Office.

Taylor, M. (2001) *Homecare. The Forgotten Service: Report on UNISON'S Survey of Home Care Workers in the UK.* London: UNISON.

TOPSS England (2000) *Modernising the Social Care Workforce: The First National Training Strategy for England.* Leeds: TOPSS England.

Trojan, L. and Yonge, O. (1993) 'Developing trusting, caring relationships: home care nurses and elderly clients.' *Journal of Advanced Nursing 18*, 1903–1910.

Twigg, J. (2000) *Bathing – The Body and Community Care.* London: Routledge.

UNISON (2003) *Working for Local Communities: A UNISON Briefing for the NJC Local Government Pay Commission April 2003*. London: UNISON.

Walmsley, J. (1998) 'Accounts of care and caring – an introduction.' In M. Alliott and M. Robb (eds) *Understanding Health and Social Care: An Introductory Reader*. Milton Keynes: Open University Press.

Webb, S., Moriarty, J. and Levin, E. (1998) *Research on Community Care: Social Work and Community Care and Community Care Arrangements for Older People with Dementia*. London: National Institute for Social Work Research Unit.

PART 2

Marginalised Socio-Cultural Issues in Dementia

The Role of Spirituality in Providing Care to Dependent Elders among African American Family Caregivers

Peggye Dilworth-Anderson

Introduction

The majority of current research on spirituality and health/well-being indicates that a positive relationship exists between the two, with individuals who report higher levels of spirituality also reporting better health (Ellison 1994; Koenig, Kvale and Ferrel 1988; Krause and Van Tran 1989; Levin, Taylor and Chatters 1995; Musick 1996; Walls and Zarit 1991; Wilson-Ford 1992). In addition, religious involvement seems to offset the negative impact of stressful life events (Krause and Van Tran 1989). Levin, Chatters and Taylor (1995), in their study of the effects of religion on health status and life satisfaction, found that individuals who perceived themselves as religious had greater life satisfaction. Similarly, Koenig *et al.* (1988) found that the more religiously oriented the elderly person was, the less agitation, dissatisfaction and greater overall morale he or she experienced.

The benefits of spirituality may be particularly significant on the health/ well-being of African Americans, and more so for African American women than men. This may be due to the high degree of spirituality exhibited by African Americans (Levin and Taylor 1993). African Americans as a group are highly involved in religious activities ·and describe themselves as very religious (Taylor 1986); however, African American women exhibit a higher degree of religiosity than African American men (Brown, Ndubuisi and Gary 1990; Koenig *et al.* 1988; Levin, Taylor and Chatters 1995). In a study examining the health-protective behaviours among black elderly women, Wilson-Ford (1992) found that more than 90 per cent of the respondents in her study used relaxation, prayer or the act of living by religious principles to protect their health. Increased religiosity has been found to be associated with less depression and physical disability among women (Mattis 2002).

Another factor contributing to the benefits that African Americans receive from spiritual beliefs and religious participation is the African American church. For many African Americans, the church provides a source of informal assistance that may contribute to feelings of well-being. Taylor and Chatters (1986) found that six out of ten persons in their study received some form of assistance from their church. Also in support of this argument, Walls and Zarit (1991) found that church support contributed to feelings of well-being among older blacks.

The purpose of this chapter is to discuss the role of religion and spirituality in assisting with caregiving among African American caregivers caring for older relatives who are both physically and cognitively impaired, and who may be at risk of dementia. It has been suggested that caring for a relative with dementia may be one of the most demanding situations encountered by caregivers (Hooker et al. 1998; Ory et al. 1999). They report that the unpredictability, duration and ambiguity associated with caregiving for a cognitively impaired relative can be very stressful for caregivers. Increasing evidence, especially the work of Koenig and colleagues (Koenig, Larson and McCullough 2001), provides insight into how caregivers may use religion and spirituality to help them cope with and respond to the stresses of caregiving to older relatives with cognitive impairment or dementia.

According to Koenig *et al.* (1988), religiosity, or one's degree of religiousness, can be manifested in three ways: organisational activity, non-organisational activity and intrinsic religiosity. Organisational activity includes frequency of attendance to one's place of worship. Non-organisational activity includes participating in religious activities that occur outside of one's place of worship, such as watching religious programmes on television or participating in spiritual activities. Intrinsic religiosity includes one's attitudes and beliefs that frame one's spiritual feelings. In all, religion entails organised and formalised systems of belief, faith and worship. Spirituality, on the other hand, is not formalised, but internally controlled by each individual. One may be both spiritual and religious, but one does not have to be religious in order to exhibit spirituality. Koenig *et al.* (2001) also suggest spirituality is more encompassing than the term religion. Spirituality can be conceived as the umbrella concept under which one finds religion and the needs of the human spirit.

When studying caregivers, it is important to distinguish between these two terms because the caregivers may or may not participate in organised religious activity such as frequent church attendance, but perceive themselves as possessing a high degree of spirituality. Consequently, this chapter seeks to explain the role that both spirituality and religiosity play in helping African American caregivers in their caregiving role.

Four questions guided this qualitative study:

1.   To what extent did caregivers identify with an organised religion?

2.   Were caregivers involved in different types of religious activities?

3.   Did the place of religion provide help to caregivers and, if so, what type of help did they receive?

4.   How much did spiritual beliefs help in providing care to the care recipient? If caregivers answered that they helped, they were then asked to describe how their spiritual beliefs have helped.

Theoretical overview

The theory of symbolic interactionism was used to guide this chapter. Symbolic interactionism posits that humans exist in a world composed of both physical and symbolic realities. Three basic premises underlie symbolic interactionism. First, people act toward objects based on the meaning those objects have for them. Second, objects are given meaning through social interaction. Third, an interpretative process takes place through which individuals handle and modify meanings based on the circumstances of a given situation (Blumer 1969). These premises are experienced within socio-culturally appropriate contexts that provide socially and culturally prescribed normative behaviours and the subjective meanings that individuals attach to these behaviours. Collectively, these subjective meanings become normalised and are shared by members in a group to help define and interpret situations, and help understand how to respond or react to them.

Meaning and definitions assigned to caregiving for African Americans are rooted in some of the spiritual beliefs shared by many African Americans.

These shared beliefs include:

1. the belief that circumstances will eventually improve because God is in control

2. the belief that those who suffer will be rewarded one day

3. the belief that one should honour one's mother and father.

(Lincoln and Mamiya 1990)

Caregiving duties such as caring for those in need, accepting caregiving obligations, and sacrificing one's time, resources and quality of life to provide for the care recipient are also Christian duties and part of the African American religious identity. Biblical scripture that requires one to 'Do unto others as you would have them do unto you' provides caregivers with an impetus for providing care to those who cared for them when they were younger. The scripture extolling Christians to 'Honour thy mother and father' also reinforces the necessity of fulfilling caregiving duties to care recipients, who are usually parents of the caregivers.

By following these religious principles, the caregiver is also fulfilling fundamental caregiving duties. However, symbolic interactionism suggests that the meaning that African American caregivers prescribe to these behaviours transcends performing everyday caregiving duties and takes on the nature of fulfilling spiritual duties. The reward of becoming a good Christian by fulfilling caregiving obligations may evoke the positive feelings of gratification that many African American caregivers report receiving from their caregiving roles. By allowing the fulfilment of their caregiving duties to assume a higher spiritual meaning, African American caregivers avoid perceiving their caregiving role as straining, depressive and insurmountable. Instead, they use their spiritual beliefs as a foundation of strength and use this strength as a resource for fulfilling their caregiving obligations.

Methods

Sampling procedures

The study participants were 187 primary, 79 secondary, 49 tertiary caregivers and 15 tertiary-only caregivers for older family members with functional and/or cognitive impairment (the care recipients in this study). Caregivers were selected in a four-stage process.

STAGE ONE

Care recipients were selected from the African American sample members of the Duke Established Populations for Epidemiological Studies of the Elderly (EPESE). The Duke EPESE is a longitudinal study with a stratified random sample of 4162 (54% African American; n=2261) non-institutionalised older persons aged 65 or older living in five contiguous counties in the Piedmont area of North Carolina (Cornoni-Huntley *et al.* 1990).

STAGE TWO

Because we wanted to use the latest available information on the potential respondents, the sample of care recipients was restricted to African American EPESE participants meeting criteria for functional and/or cognitive impairment at the follow-up interview six years after baseline. Criteria for selection were: inability to perform two or more basic activities of daily living (Branch *et al.* 1984) and/or a score of three or more on the Short Portable Mental Status Questionnaire (SPMSQ), and a brief screen of cognitive functioning (Pfeiffer 1975). This reduced the sample size to 497.

STAGE THREE

Of the 497 African American elderly in the EPESE study who met the above criteria, 31 per cent had died, nine per cent had been institutionalised, four per cent could not be contacted, three per cent refused to participate, and six per cent had no caregiver when this study began in 1995. This resulted in a sample of 234 elderly African Americans who were eligible for the study. The EPESE study (1992–1993) provided information on socio-demographic characteristics, physical health status, level of cognitive impairment, and ability to perform activities of daily living for this group of 234 elderly.

STAGE FOUR

Letters were sent to all eligible participants (n=234). Some of the elderly participants could be contacted directly (n=124) and others were contacted via a proxy (n=110). The letters informed them of our study and how we obtained their names, addresses and phone numbers. A follow-up telephone call was made to schedule a time for a short telephone interview. This screening telephone interview with the elderly participants or a proxy respondent was conducted to determine if they had a primary person who helped provide them with care and support. Once identified, this person was contacted by phone to determine specific caregiving roles and responsibilities, and an interview was scheduled. Ten per cent of the 234 caregivers refused to participate, two per cent could not be contacted, and two per cent of the care recipients had died or were institutionalised. As a result, our sample comprised 202 caregivers. Fifteen of these caregivers provided limited specialised support and were not included in this study. The other 187 were primary caregivers and had main responsibilities and/or provided the most care for the care recipient. Interviews were conducted with all 187 primary caregivers, 79 secondary, 49 tertiary and 15 tertiary-only caregivers. Because this analysis focuses on caregivers that provided the most care, this study includes only primary, secondary and tertiary caregivers. Findings are also reported according to caregiving structures that include a combination of caregivers. These structures include the following combinations: primary-only; primary, secondary and tertiary; primary and secondary; and primary and tertiary (Dilworth-Anderson, Williams and Cooper 1999).

Data analysis

Qualitative data from the open-ended questions were analysed using thematic analysis. Thematic analysis can help to uncover concepts, values and processes not captured by standardised measures as administered through structured interviews. 'Themes can provide insight into the cultural beliefs and values that instil powerful experiences and motivations, and shape how individuals plan, make sense of, and respond to events' (Luborsky 1994, p.190). Luborsky (p.195) defined themes as broad, overarching statements by informants that directly reflect their values, beliefs and commitments. This definition 'helps to provide a clear orientation to work that seeks to understand and reflect the informant's own views and words'.

Several steps were involved in the thematic analysis of the data. First, each text file from the caregiver interview was read in its entirety by four trained researchers. Next, open coding was conducted which allows a researcher to provisionally formulate concepts and categories that seem to fit the data (Strauss and Corbin 1990). Having read each transcript once, readers developed a consensus on the codes identified on the role spirituality played in their caregiving role and how spirituality helped carers in their role.

Second, further coding of the data was used to determine whether subcategories were inclusive within the larger themes already identified. During the second step, this phase of coding is called axial coding. Axial coding is a more directed form of open coding that consists of intense analysis done around one category (what we call a domain) at a time. Knowledge about relationships between a category/domain and other categories and subcategories provides more cumulative information on a topic (Strauss and Corbin 1990).

From this process, data was coded to fit specific domains created from the initial coding process, and then several smaller themes that fit into the domain constructed were added for a better understanding of the domain.

The domains were listed and described in detail with several direct quotes from the caregivers taken directly from the transcripts to represent each theme. Data management and coding were undertaken using the Ethnograph version 4.0 computer program for analysing, coding and quantifying qualitative data. The Ethnograph program confirmed four major domains emergent in the caregivers' text responses that were in accordance with the following criteria:

1. Strength – respondents indicated that their spiritual beliefs provided them with some form of strength that assisted them in their caregiving duties.

2. Duty/Reciprocity – respondents indicated that they viewed caregiving as their duty and/or they expected to receive caregiving for themselves during times of need.

3. Faith – respondents indicated that acts such as praying, having faith in God, and believing that God was in control of their lives enabled them to perform their caregiving duties.

4. Gratification – respondents indicated receiving positive feelings such as joy, love and fulfilment from the process of caregiving.

Findings

QUESTIONS 1 AND 2

These two questions addressed religious affiliation and the level of involvement in different types of religious activities. Analysis shows that 96 per cent of all caregivers in this study are Christian and are active in organised and non-organised activities such as attending church (89%), watching religious services on the television, and listening to religious programming (66%). The most popular activities are missionary group (33–75%), Bible study (42–50%) and prayer meetings (28–50%). Tertiary-only caregivers were more active than the other caregivers, but their activities seem to correspond with the duties they performed as caregivers: infrequent and less demanding of their time.

QUESTION 3

This question allowed for assessing the extent to which caregivers' place of religion provided help and, if so, the type of help they received. Most caregivers (78–93%) felt they received no help with caregiving from their place of worship. The caregivers who felt they received support from their place of worship (2–15%) believed people in the church prayed for them, gave them advice and encouragement, sent spiritual leaders or personally visited, and sent food at least once a month. Secondary caregivers reported receiving financial assistance on occasion (50%). The church members rarely provided transportation for any of the caregivers. Among the few caregivers that did receive this assistance, it was provided inconsistently (primary caregiver 17%, secondary caregiver 13%).

QUESTION 4

The extent to which spirituality helped caregivers and their perceptions of how spirituality helped them to provide care to their dependent elderly family members were addressed in this question. The responses among those caregivers who were asked this question are included in the findings reported here. A total of 186 primary caregivers responded: 156 said that spiritual beliefs helped a lot, 21 said their beliefs helped somewhat or a little, and nine said that their spiritual beliefs did not help at all. A total of 62 secondary caregivers responded: 53 said that spiritual beliefs helped a lot, six said their beliefs helped somewhat or a little, and three said that their spiritual beliefs did not help at all. A total of 46 tertiary caregivers responded: 36 said that spiritual beliefs helped a lot, six said their beliefs helped somewhat or a little, and four said that their spiritual beliefs did not help at all.

Almost half (45%) of the caregivers reported that their spirituality gave them strength, courage, patience and peace of mind in performing their caregiving duties and responsibilities. Twenty-four per cent of caregivers indicated that some form of faith (e.g. identifying God as having control over the outcomes of their lives or praying) assisted them in caregiving activities. Duty and reciprocity, the giving back to those who care for us and living up to Christian duties by caring for one's mother and father, were identified by 24 per cent of the caregivers. Finally, seven per cent of all caregivers indicated experiencing some form of gratification or positive feelings through the performance of their caregiving roles (see Figure 4.1).

Using open-ended questions, information was gathered on caregivers' perceptions of how their spirituality helped them to provide care to their dependent elderly family members. The findings reported below reflect care-

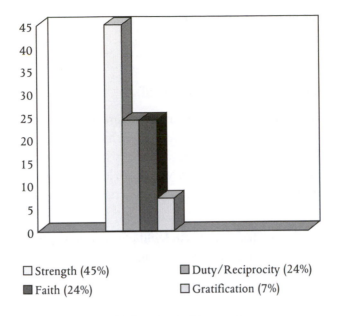

Strength (45%)   Duty/Reciprocity (24%)
Faith (24%)   Gratification (7%)

Figure 4.1 Domains of spiritual help indentified by caregivers

givers providing care to elders who have physical health problems, those that are cognitively impaired, or the combination of both. These responses, called text responses, were analysed according to individual caregivers and caregiving structures as discussed earlier, and consisted of different types of caregivers. Four themes were identified with the most common themes being Strength and Duty/Reciprocity. Many caregivers indicated similar variations of their belief, and that their spiritual beliefs allowed them to persevere in their caregiving roles. A significant number of individuals in the caregiving structures also indicated that their spiritual beliefs gave them moral guidelines for behaviour, including caregiving responsibilities.

Below are some examples of the text responses provided by individuals in various caregiving structures. Caregivers responded to the question: 'How have your spiritual beliefs helped?' Responses to this question are included below.

The participants from the first caregiving structure consisted of a primary (PR) and a secondary (SE) caregiver caring for an older relative who was cognitively impaired, and was described as having memory problems by caregivers. It is possible that this older relative may have had some form of dementia. Each respondent indicated very clearly that their spiritual beliefs gave them strength.

'HOW HAVE YOUR SPIRITUAL BELIEFS HELPED?'

Domain on strength

0078 PR Made me stronger.

0078 SE Stronger faith in God and myself.

The participants from the next caregiving structure also indicated that they derived strength from their spiritual beliefs, but in more salient terms than the first group. This caregiving structure also consisted of a primary and a secondary caregiver caring for a relative with high levels of both physical and cognitive impairment, and who may have been at risk of having some form of dementia.

0172 PR No matter what you do, God will give you strength. All things happen for a reason. All my strength comes from God.

0172 SE When I'm down I'm uplifted. The more I read the Bible the stronger I get.

The next caregiving structure consisted of a primary, secondary and tertiary (TE) caregiver. In this instance only the primary and secondary caregivers' responses reflected similar themes of strength.

0476 PR Strong faith in God. When you don't feel like going on, faith provides strength.

0476 SE Keeps me strong and going [belief in God].

0476 TE Helps me believe I'm doing the right thing by helping out.

Domain on duty and reciprocity

As stated earlier, another common theme among caregiving structures was the belief that spiritual beliefs provided moral or religious guidelines for behaviour regarding their caregiving duties and responsibilities. An example of this belief can be found in the following text responses taken from a primary and secondary caregiver caring for an older relative with high levels of both physical and cognitive impairment, and who may have been at risk of having some form of dementia.

The secondary caregiver from this structure clearly indicates that her spirituality provided guidelines for treating one's parents, as found in the scriptures (Bible).

0217 PR If angry, being a Christian helps your attitude towards other people and your parents.

0217 SE   Understanding from a scripture standpoint what Jehovah expects. How we should treat our parents.

A second example of the moral guidelines derived from spiritual beliefs is illustrated below. Interestingly, both respondents quoted the Biblical phrase 'Honour thy mother and father' and applied it to their caregiving responsibilities.

0337 PR   Honour thy father and mother. Mom took care of me when I could not do for myself so I will do everything possible in her time of need.

0337 TE   I've always been taught to honour your father and mother and watched parents care for others in family and I was taught to do this.

The final caregiving structure for this theme of duty and reciprocity consisted of a primary, secondary and tertiary caregiver. Although the primary caregivers indicated that spirituality made them strong and gave them peace of mind, the secondary and tertiary caregivers both indicated deriving guidelines for behaviour from their spiritual beliefs. Again, the use of Bible quotes is quite common in these responses. The secondary caregiver uses two, in fact, and relates both quotes directly to her caregiving responsibilities.

0484 PR   Keeps him strong; more attentive with her. Keeps him from stressing out and [helps him] not to worry.

0484 SE   Believe in the Bible teaching, 'Thou should honour your mother and father.' Jesus teaches us to love one another. She thinks of parents as children and Jesus says, 'Suffer the little children to come unto me.'

0484 TE   I believe in God; God is love. I love my mother. The Bible quotes 'honour thy mother and father'.

Domain on faith
The theme of faith was also important in how caregivers' sense of spirituality helped them with their caregiving. A caregiver made the following statement caring for an older relative with a high level of cognitive impairment, and who may have been at risk of some form of dementia. She indicated that, basically, she provided care alone. She was not in a caregiver structure that included a major secondary or tertiary caregiver that provided help to her.

0554 PR   When you don't feel like going on, faith provides strength.

The next set of statements about faith represents caregivers in a primary, secondary and tertiary caregiving structure.

0022 PR   My faith keeps me strong; keeps me from stressing out and not to worry.

0022 SE   Knowing from the Bible that right rules over wrong, it inspires me to do for my mother.

0022 TE   God will provide.

Domain on gratification

Caregivers also indicated that they derived positive feelings or gratification from performing their caregiving roles, as indicated by text responses from the following caregivers caring for an older relative with high levels of both physical and cognitive impairment, and who may have been at risk of having some form of dementia.

These responses came from a primary and secondary caregiver caring for an older relative with both physical and cognitive impairments.

0553 PR   Just having a feeling of fulfilment, helpfulness and thankfulness that she is as well as she is. Gave me encouragement and peace of mind.

0553 SE   It helped me – like a blessing to help someone that has taken care of you. Best to give than to receive and I feel good about it.

Summary and discussion

Guided by symbolic interaction theory, the purpose of this chapter was to discuss the role of religion and spirituality in assisting with caregiving among African American caregivers. The key concepts of meanings, definitions and interpretations from symbolic interaction provided conceptual direction for analysing the responses provided by African American caregivers (Blumer 1969). Symbolic interaction, therefore, was used to provide conceptual direction for interpreting shared beliefs or lack of them among the caregivers caring for dependent elders in their families who often had both cognitive and physical limitations. Although the data collected on the care recipients used in this study was not specific to dementia they did provide a level of understanding on caring for older care recipients with cognitive impairments. There is evidence that points to levels of cognitive impairments providing a window into understanding the effect of providing care to older relatives who eventually become demented (Dilworth-Anderson, Williams and Gibson 2002).

Of interest in this study was the understanding of how different caregivers, in what we describe as structures of care, gave meanings to their roles in relation to their spiritual beliefs. The study was also able to provide more quantitative data on religious affiliations and activities.

Our findings also demonstrate that:

- the majority of caregivers did participate in religious activities

- the majority of caregivers did not receive help with their caregiving roles from their place of worship

- the majority of caregivers reported that their spirituality assisted them with their caregiving duties

- spirituality gave caregivers strength, a sense of duty and feelings of 'giving back', faith and gratification.

An important finding noted here is that although the majority of caregivers were affiliated with a place of religion, they received very little support from the church. Nevertheless, caregivers were overwhelmingly rooted in strong spiritual beliefs. Their caregiving was, therefore, more strongly supported by their spirituality than informal support from their place of religion.

Our findings show that spirituality assisted caregivers by giving them strength; it defined and reinforced their Christian duties of honouring their mothers and fathers by giving back to them the care that they had received when young. It also gave them the faith that they could 'carry on', and it provided them with a sense of gratification and a positive attitude that they had fulfilled their roles to their dependent parents. Another important finding was that the majority of caregivers in their respective families, as indicated by caregiving structures, had shared meanings about the role of spirituality in helping them as caregivers. Several inferences and interpretations can be made from this finding. First, these shared meanings can be interpreted as caregivers having shared perceived benefits from their spiritual beliefs. One of the benefits of spirituality is that it can serve as a health-protective barrier against negative health outcomes and it can prolong survival (Helm *et al.* 2000; Strawbridge *et al.* 2001). This finding also suggests that when different caregivers in the same family share strong spiritual beliefs about their caregiving, they are less likely to experience role conflict and possibly feelings of burden or stress. Most importantly, this finding of shared spiritual beliefs and caregiving shows that African American caregivers have given meaning to their sense of coping – it is spiritual. This spiritual way of coping with caregiving may serve to help interpret the consistent finding in the literature that African American caregivers experience less depression than is found among their white counterparts (Dilworth-Anderson *et al.* 2002).

Notwithstanding some of the positive findings reported in this chapter, a note of caution needs to be made. African American caregivers still under-utilise formal care which might help reinforce the high level of informal care family caregivers provide; care that is obviously supported by strong spiritual beliefs. A marked problem in providing assistance to African American caregivers is their traditional reluctance to use formal assistance. Although the church provided a low level of support to the caregivers in our study, we believe that the black church can serve as a bridge through which African American caregivers can have access to formal services. By working with local churches, formal service agencies can gain credibility in the eyes of African American caregivers, and so will facilitate access to the African American community and its caregivers. With outside assistance, these caregivers may be able to provide better care for their dependent elderly family members, and receive help for themselves. The long-term benefits of this assistance may even extend to an improved health status of the caregivers when they in turn become care recipients.

References

Blumer, H. (1969) *Symbolic Interactionism: Perspective and Method.* Englewood Cliffs, NJ: Prentice-Hall.

Branch, L.G., Katz, S., Kniepmann, K. and Papsidero, J. (1984) 'A prospective study of functional status among community elders.' *American Journal of Public Health 74,* 266–268.

Brown, D.R., Ndubuisi, S.C. and Gary, L.E. (1990) 'Religiosity and psychological distress among blacks.' *Journal of Religion and Health 29,* 1, 55–68.

Cornoni-Huntley, J., Blazer, D.G., Service, C. and Farmer, M.E. (1990) 'Introduction.' In J. Cornoni-Huntley, D.G. Blazer, M.E. Lafferty, D.F. Everett, D.B. Brock and M.E. Farmer (eds) *Established Populations for Epidemiologic Studies of the Elderly, Volume II: Resource Data Book.* Washington, DC: NIH Publication No. 90–495.

Dilworth-Anderson, P., Williams, I.C. and Gibson, B.E. (2002) 'Issues of race, ethnicity, and culture in caregiving research: a twenty-year review (1980–2000).' *The Gerontologist 42,* 327–272.

Dilworth-Anderson, P., Williams, S.W. and Cooper, T. (1999) 'Family caregiving to elderly African Americans: caregiver types and structures.' *Journal of Gerontology: Social Sciences 54,* 237–341.

Ellison, C.G. (1994) 'Religion, the life stress paradigm and the study of depression.' In J. Levin (ed) *Religion in Ageing and Health.* Thousand Oaks, CA: Sage Publications.

Helm, H.M., Hays, J.C., Flint, E.P., Koenig, H.G. and Blazer, D.G. (2000) 'Does private religious activity prolong survival? A six-year follow-up study of 3851 older adults.' *Journals of Gerontology Series A: Biological Sciences and Medical Sciences 55,* M400–M405.

Hooker, K., Monahan, D.J., Bowman, S.R., Frazier, L.D. and Shifren, K. (1998) 'Personality counts for a lot: predictors of mental and physical health of spouse caregivers in two disease groups.' *Journal of Gerontology Series B: Social Sciences 53*, P73–P85.

Koenig, H., Kvale, J. and Ferrel, C. (1988) 'Religion and well-being in later life.' *The Gerontologist 28*, 18–28.

Koenig, H.G., Larson, D.B. and McCullough, M.E. (2001) *Handbook of Religion and Health*. New York: Oxford University Press.

Krause, N. and Van Tran, T. (1989) 'Stress and religious involvement among older blacks.' *Journal of Gerontology: Social Sciences 44*, 1, S4–S13.

Levin, J.S. and Taylor, R.J. (1993) 'Gender and age differences in religiosity among Black Americans.' *The Gerontologist 33*, 1, 16–23.

Levin, J., Chatters, L. and Taylor, R. (1995) 'Religious effects on health status and life satisfaction among Americans.' *Journal of Gerontology: Social Sciences 50B*, S154–S163.

Levin, J.S., Taylor, R.J. and Chatters, L.M. (1995) 'A multidimensional measure of religious involvement for African Americans.' *The Sociological Quarterly 36*, 1, 157–173.

Lincoln, C.E. and Mamiya, L.H. (1990) *The Black Church in the African American Experience*. Durham, NC: Duke University Press.

Luborsky, M. (1994) 'The identification and analysis of themes and patterns.' In J.F. Gubrium and A. Sankar (eds) *Qualitative Methods in Ageing Research*. Thousand Oaks, CA: Sage Publications.

Mattis, J.S. (2002) 'The role of religion and spirituality in the coping experience of African American women: a qualitative analysis.' *Psychology of Women Quarterly 26*, 308–320.

Musick, M. (1996) 'Religion and subjective health among black and white elderly.' *Journal of Health and Social Behaviour 37*, 221–237.

Ory, M.G., Hoffman, R.R., Yee, J.L., Tennstedt, S. and Schulz, R. (1999) 'Prevalence and impact of caregiving: a detailed comparison between dementia and non-dementia caregivers.' *The Gerontologist 39*, 177–185.

Pfeiffer, E. (1975) 'A short portable mental status questionnaire for the assessment of organic brain deficit in elderly patients.' *Journal of the American Geriatrics Society 10*, 433–441.

Strauss, A. and Corbin, J. (1990) *Basics of Qualitative Research*. Newbury Park: Sage Publications.

Strawbridge, W.J., Shema, S.J., Cohen, R.D. and Kaplan, G.A. (2001) 'Religious attendance increases survival by improving and maintaining good health behaviours, mental health, and social relationships.' *Annals of Behavioral Medicine 23*, 68–74.

Taylor, R.J. (1986) 'Religious participation among elderly Blacks.' *The Gerontologist 26*, 6, 630–636.

Taylor, R.J. and Chatters, L.M. (1986) 'Church-based informal support among elderly Blacks.' *The Gerontologist 26*, 6, 637–642.

Walls, C.T. and Zarit, S. (1991) 'Informal support from Black churches and the well-being of elderly Blacks.' *The Gerontologist 31*, 4, 490–495.

Wilson-Ford, V. (1992) 'Health-protective behaviours of rural black elderly women.' *Health and Social Work 17*, 28–36.

CHAPTER 5

Death and Dying

Sylvia Cox and Karen Watchman

Introduction

Death is claimed to be a taboo subject in modern Western societies. Death and the dying experience are often medicalised with the person who is near death removed to institutions such as hospitals and hospices. Death is usually controlled by health professionals and technology, care being provided by strangers rather than the family, and often not within a religious framework (Giddens 1991). The topic of death may be avoided in both professional and personal life (Bond and Bond 1986) but paradoxically dying and death are now more readily discussed in everyday conversation (McNamara 2001, quoting Ballard). The way that dying people and their families are responded to is likely to reflect the perceptions and social patterns that inform a particular society (McNamara 2001).

In many ways people with dementia typify the changing nature of death in modern Western societies. Death is now more likely to occur:

- in old age
- as a result of one or a number of long-term chronic illnesses
- with dying extended over months or years (often due to drug treatment and technology)
- with the certainty of death emerging slowly over a long period of time
- in hospital or care home
- with the dying cared for by staff rather than family
- with prediction of death more problematic.

In this chapter we will consider how people with dementia who are dying may be further marginalised and excluded from receiving appropriate health interventions, social care and support as they approach the end of life. We use case examples to illustrate some of the issues, reflecting situations arising from practice and development work carried out by the authors in the fields of both dementia care and learning disability.

Perspectives on dementia

Two models of disability that are often discussed as part of considering interventions when a person has dementia and is dying are the medical and social models (Oliver 1996).

The medical model has been adapted over the years to encompass more than just drugs and medication. It can be seen to cover counselling and, in some cases, alternative therapies. This is an ever-changing area with drugs now available for the early stages of dementia and research ongoing for new medication. Although not without side effects these drugs can be beneficial if administered in the early stages (Marshall 2001b). A purely medical model, dependent on a health-related intervention specifically for the person with dementia, may lead to a lack of recognition of the role of those who care for them, by not recognising or acknowledging their input.

The social model alone can also be seen to have limitations. It is an approach that considers different forms of interventions such as adaptations to the environment (Marshall 2001a) and reminiscence work (Killick and Allan 2001). The social model considers more than just the person. It takes into account where they live, who with and what activities and resources can be used for their benefit.

While the medical model may not always fully include carers or an under-standing of the person's social networks, the social model may put less emphasis on medical intervention for pain relief and alleviation of symptoms. The value for the person with dementia and their carers is to combine the best from both approaches as each on its own can be seen to have limitations.

A feared death

Cancer is often perceived as the most feared death. There are many reasons for this: it is unpredictable, dying is often painful and prolonged and people with cancer may be 'blamed' for bringing on cancer through risky behaviours, diet, smoking or sexual behaviour. There are many parallels between cancer and dementia. Like cancer, dementia is unpredictable, its causes uncertain, and drug treatment is only slowly becoming available and is not curative. Dementia differs in that it is strongly associated with actual or anticipated multiple losses: of memory, of the ability to communicate and care for oneself, of bodily functions, of home, of awareness of self, of relationships. Images and perceptions of cancer are frightening and awful but the words used to describe dementia include 'a shell', a 'living death' (Woods 1989), of becoming a nothingness, a fate worse than death.

The term 'social death' may be used to refer to the process whereby the person ceases to be a significant actor in everyday life, before biological death occurs (Sweeting 1997). Family members may feel that they have already lost their relative with dementia as the illness progresses. Depending on the type and progress of dementia the person may cease to recognise loved ones and the person themselves may seem very different from their old self. However, sometimes those caring for the person may treat the person as if they are dead, not attempting to find ways of communicating and understanding needs, thus denying their personhood. Kitwood (1997) exemplified this by 'the dementia in bed 3'.

Case example 1: Jim

Jim (81) had dementia. No discussion took place about Jim's future preferences, as the diagnosis was not shared with him. The doctor felt that there was little that could be done and it was just a matter of time. Jim also had high blood pressure and controlled late onset diabetes.

For a couple of years Jim maintained many of his interests and enjoyment of walking, bridge and listening to music continued. However, there was no real care plan and the family had to try to keep track of what was happening by phone and when they visited, which was mainly at weekends when no staff were available.

His family began to think about the need for a care home as they could see he was deteriorating rapidly. However, he suddenly collapsed and was admitted to hospital with cardiac failure. Jim hit out at a nurse who attempted to toilet him and he was sedated which made his agitation worse. There was a delay in notifying his family of his admission. When they eventually visited they were able to give information to staff about their father's preferences. However, this was not passed on when he was transferred to the rehabilitation ward.

As he was not mentioning any pain, pain relief was not given, even though he always became more agitated when being moved or touched. There was no discussion between hospital staff and family about the likely prognosis.

Two weeks later Jim was abruptly discharged from the ward. The rapid response team supported him at home for four weeks but it was clear that he needed 24-hour support and nursing care. Eventually, the family arranged a place in a care home. He moved in to the care home, where he remained in a distressed and agitated state. One night, he collapsed again and was admitted to the acute admissions ward of the hospital and died two days later.

Dying with dementia and dying with other conditions

There are some indications that people with dementia are treated differently from other groups receiving health and social care. Research in the UK comparing cancer patients with people with dementia shows that the latter experience symptoms for longer and are much more likely to have lived in residential care during their last year of life. Forty-three per cent of the study population had lived in a nursing or residential home and 41 per cent had died there. People with dementia were seen by their GP less than patients with cancer, and 67 per cent had a hospital stay during their last year with 26 per cent in hospital for more than three months (McCarthy, Addington-Hall and Altmann 1997).

Time of dying

One of the complexities is that people die at many points throughout the journey of dementia (Cox and Cook 2002). This results in a vast range of different needs and experiences, including, for example, those who have:

- a mix of acquired mental and physical problems, but where brain impairment is not advanced
- advanced dementia, and who die of the complications of dementia
- some other condition such as cancer or heart problems as well as dementia
- dementia on top of a lifelong disability such as Down's Syndrome or other types of learning disability.

Age, gender, disability, culture, ethnic background, and mental and physical health will affect expressed needs. Thus a man in his 50s with early onset

Alzheimer's disease may be much more concerned about his diagnosis of lung cancer than the impact of dementia. Some research exists about the 'end stages' of dementia (Coetzee, Leask and Jones 2003; Luchins and Hanrahan 1995). Studies have tended to focus on specific interventions without looking at palliative care as an overall approach. This is an area where relatively little research has been carried out, especially in the UK.

Although dementia mostly affects people in their later years, smaller numbers of younger people are also affected. One of these groups is people with learning disability, especially those with Down's Syndrome.

People with Down's Syndrome are living for longer and it is known that they are developing dementia at a younger age than the general population. Literature and research are significantly lacking when considering end of life issues for people with Down's Syndrome and dementia. There is still debate about whether people with dementia should be informed of their diagnosis (Downs 2000), although increasingly good practice involves sharing the diagnosis in a supportive way. However, many people with Down's Syndrome are not even aware that they have a learning disability. People with Down's Syndrome are often not told if dementia is diagnosed, and in some cases nor are their carers. This has been recorded as due to health professionals not wanting to increase the stress experienced by family members who already have a caring role (Watchman 2003). This precludes them from choosing to take part in any form of care at the end of their life especially if it is not made clear to them, or their family, that the disease they have may be terminal.

Case example 2: Lynne

Lynne (50) has Down's Syndrome and dementia. Lynne lives in a supported accommodation project with 22 other adults with a learning disability. Lynne has had no contact with any of her family for 40 years.

Lynne can no longer climb the stairs to bed at night. Every evening a staff member takes her in a taxi to a nearby nursing home, where she sleeps in a ground floor bedroom. She is taxied back to the supported accommodation project again the next morning.

Staff in the supported accommodation project do not feel that Lynne should continue to live there, despite it being her home for 17 years, as they do not know anything about dementia. Staff at the nursing home do not feel that she should stay there, as they do not know anything about Down's Syndrome.

While neither staff group are willing to listen to and learn from each other, equally important is that neither staff group are taking into account that Lynne has serious health issues. As an older person with Down's Syndrome she is prone to other health problems such as hypothyroidism, depression and loss of sight and hearing, in addition to the dementia that is known about.

Lynne is unable to communicate verbally to staff so cannot indicate pain, discomfort, distress or hunger other than by gesture or action, often resulting in staff labelling her behaviour as 'a problem'.

Terminal or palliative care

There is an increasing emphasis on early diagnosis, availability of drug treatment and other interventions to maximise quality of life for people with dementia. This raises questions about the appropriateness of referring to dementia as a terminal condition, although unless another condition intervenes it will be so. The term 'palliative care' may thus be used in both general and specific ways. Palliative care may now be applied to all life-limiting conditions, though is still most strongly associated with cancer (McCarthy *et al.* 1997). The generally accepted view of palliative care dates back to 1990 and the World Health Organisation. This stated that palliative care would improve the quality of life of patients and their families when one of their members had a life-threatening illness. This would be achieved through the prevention and relief of suffering by assessing and treating pain. It would also work with non-medical problems such as those of an emotional, social and spiritual nature. The palliative care process was to be viewed as a 'normal process' (World Health Organisation 1990) and would offer support to patients and their families not just at the final stages of their illness, but throughout its course, and for the duration of the bereavement process. Palliative care approaches do not appear to be widely available in the community, care homes and hospitals (Evers *et al.* 2002).

Barriers to providing specialist palliative care to people with dementia in the UK, even those with cancer, are identified (NCHSPCS and SPAPCC 2000). The reasons proposed include:

- problems in diagnosis
- dementia not being recognised as a terminal illness
- problems in predicting life expectancy and thus the dying trajectory

- concerns about the levels of challenging behaviour in people with dementia

- perceived inability of people with dementia to know that they are dying and therefore being less able to enter into a therapeutic relationship.

Some of these perceived 'problems' of caring for people with dementia who are dying have been evidenced in the first two case studies. For example, Jim and Lynne experience problems in having their condition recognised and understood. Constantly being moved to different locations means that their need for continuity and familiar people and places is ignored. Because communication is a problem, efforts to find different ways of understanding need, especially pain and intimate care, are not engaged. This results in their marginalisation and exclusion from the process of planning for their death.

A different approach

The person-centred approach to dementia care puts people at the centre and proposes positive approaches to improve quality of life (Kitwood 1997). This person-centred approach to care sets out a value base that is focused on the worth and dignity of all human beings and affirms their uniqueness and individuality regardless of age, disability or illness (Kitwood 1997). Human dignity includes the dignity of the body – 'one's living body is intrinsic to one's personhood' (Finnis 1992, p.194) – and so may oppose the processes of social death and exclusion.

Palliative care is rarely a person-centred experience for people with dementia, as the focus by professionals and family members often remains on specific aspects of the disease, such as memory loss, rather than seeing the palliative care process as beginning with the diagnosis of dementia.

The way that others – professionals, family and friends – respond to needs may be governed by the expectations about dementia, so that autonomy is denied. One aspect of autonomy is the person's involvement in the decision-making process. This means that ideally the person with dementia is given a choice over how their future needs are met. Addington-Hall (2002) raises the ethical question of how death with autonomy can be achieved if carers are not of the same opinion as the person who is dying. As the family unit is often central to caring for a dying relative, the autonomy of the individual may not be as evident. There is also the possibility that health professionals may impose their own views, based on different criteria such as resources, cost and personal opinion, thus reducing the autonomy of the individual. Determining the capacity of the person to give consent is crucial to retaining their autonomy and ensuring their inclusion in any decisions made about themselves. Decisions made early in the course of the illness need to be respected even as capacity decreases.

Case example 3: Brian

Brian had Down's Syndrome and dementia. The diagnosis was shared with both Brian himself and his sister Dorothy. Brian lives in a supported accommodation project with 24-hour staff support.

Dorothy found out as much as she could about dementia. Armed with literature, she asked for a case conference to be called to specifically discuss Brian's future care.

As a result of this, and after discussions with Brian, he remained in his home, although a number of changes were made. Staff received training in dementia care, as did the other tenants in the home. This meant that they were aware of the reasons for the changes in Brian's behaviour.

Nursing staff were brought in to cater for Brian's medical needs and worked alongside the residential staff over a period of months. Both later acknowledged how much they had learnt from the other.

As is often the case with people with Down's Syndrome, Brian's dementia progressed rapidly. He developed epilepsy and required 24-hour nursing. This continued in an environment that was familiar, among faces that were also familiar.

Brian died of pneumonia aged 46, two years after he was diagnosed with dementia.

Without his sister's insistence that they were both involved in his future care planning, Brian's care may have been very different in his final months. By listening to his family, Brian's care was centred around his individual needs based on his own wishes. Brian's physical and emotional needs were met as he died and both he and his family were included in the process.

Case example 4: Jane

Jane was in her late 70s when diagnosed with Alzheimer's disease. Her GP shared the diagnosis with her and discussed with her what the future may hold. Her family were aware of her desire to die at home rather than be admitted to hospital.

After a very slow gentle decline, Jane suddenly deteriorated and became too frail to leave her bed. At one stage, although she had mainly lost the power of speech, she began to cry out and say prayer words. Although she had not gone to church for many years she seemed much comforted when the local priest came and prayed with her.

A more detailed care plan was drawn up with the district nurses, home carer nightsitter and family. Her GP confirmed that the goal of care was to maximise comfort and that drugs would cease except for analgesics. The family were clear that hospitalisation was to be avoided if at all possible.

Mouth care, pressure care and continence management was continued as set out in the care plan. Comfort measures such as playing music tapes and gentle hand massage were given.

Friends and family came to sit with Jane frequently. Family members wanted to be included in the physical care, and were shown how to manage some of the care procedures such as pressure sore care.

Jane died peacefully in her sleep a week after contracting pneumonia. She died in her own bed with her husband and children by her side.

The experiences of Brian and Jane show how people with dementia, including those with other conditions such as Down's Syndrome, can be included in the process of dying. There was an acknowledgement of dementia as a terminal illness and the process of care focused on Brian and Jane as individuals rather than as Jim and Lynne who were dependent on services and available resources. This meant that their choices and preferences were both informed and meaningful. Consistency of care was important in both cases, with control over pain relief and access to other interventions available to them both as appropriate.

Involving professional and frontline staff

'Basic' palliative care (NHS Scotland 2002) aims at ensuring that care delivery is performed with a palliative care approach across all aspects of healthcare among all professionals. However, it is not always the case that people with dementia, or Down's Syndrome and dementia, are being cared for by health professionals. They are often not even known to health professionals during the early stages of the disease (Wilkinson and Janicki 2002). Many continue to live and be cared for in the family home, or in a supported accommodation environment, by informal and formal carers who do not have any health training.

In specialist dementia care units staff will regularly share information with patients and their families and discuss appropriate care. In many nursing homes, or supported accommodation projects for people with a learning disability, staff receive training and support only in relation to their specific client group. Rarely will staff working with older people receive training or information on working with people with learning disabilities. Staff in supported accommodation projects or home care will rarely receive training on dementia care. Yet an increasingly ageing population, with and without learning disabilities, suggests that this would increase the likelihood of staff understanding the needs of a diverse range of people with individual health, social and spiritual needs. Greater understanding and knowledge would enable greater consistency of care rather than staff feeling that they are unable to work with the person who has dementia.

Conclusion

A number of issues have been raised that highlight how people with dementia are both marginalised and excluded from the decision-making process when they are dying. Bringing together person-centred approaches with holistic palliative care approaches may be one way to develop more appropriate, better informed and skilled models of care. In seeking to learn from examples of social exclusion and marginalisation we suggest that joint health and social care policy and practice may be improved, leading to a more inclusive approach to the final phase of caring for people with dementia.

In order to reverse this situation there needs to be an acknowledgement that 'death' is not simply a medical term controlled by health professionals and used to describe the last stages of a person's life. Improving communication between professionals, people with dementia and carers that puts the person with dementia and their future wishes for themselves as central is essential.

Professionals, people with dementia and carers need to be included in any policy making or development of guidelines for the end of life of people with dementia.

The experience of Jim and Lynne reinforces marginalisation and reminds us only too clearly how much work remains to be done in this area. The situation of Jane and Brian, bringing in medical, social and spiritual interventions at all stages, demonstrates that the inclusion of people with dementia in determining their own care and future planning is both real and successful. It is this model that should continue to be developed.

References

Addington-Hall, J. (2002) 'Research sensitivities to palliative care patients.' *European Journal of Cancer Care 11*, 3, 220–224.

Bond, J. and Bond, S. (1986) *Sociology and Health Care: An Introduction for Nurses and Other Health Care Professionals.* Edinburgh: Churchill Livingstone.

Coetzee, R.H., Leask, S.J. and Jones, R.G. (2003) 'The attitude of carers and old age psychiatrists towards the treatment of potentially fatal events in end stage dementia.' *International Journal of Geriatric Psychiatry 18*, 2, 169–173.

Cox, S. and Cook, A. (2002) 'Caring for people with dementia at the end of life.' In J. Hockley and D. Clark (eds) *Palliative Care for Older People in Care Homes.* Buckingham: Open University Press.

Downs, M. (2000) 'Dementia in a socio-cultural context: an idea whose time has come.' *Ageing and Society 20*, 3, 369–375.

Evers, M.M., Purohit, D., Perl, D., Khan, K. and Martin, D.B. (2002) 'Palliative care and aggressive end of life care for patients with dementia.' *Psychiatric Services 5395*, 609–661.

Finnis, J. (1992) 'Economics, justice and the value of life.' In L. Gormally (ed) *The Dependent Elderly: Autonomy, Justice and Quality of Care.* Cambridge: Cambridge University Press.

Giddens, A. (1991) *Modernity and Self Identity.* Cambridge: Polity.

Killick, J. and Allan, K. (2001) *Communication and the Care of People with Dementia.* Buckingham: Open University Press.

Kitwood, T. (1997) *Dementia Reconsidered: The Person Comes First.* Buckingham: Open University Press.

Luchins, D. and Hanrahan, P. (1995) 'Access to hospice programmes in end stage dementia: a national survey of hospice programmes.' *Journal of American Geriatric Society 8*, 155–164.

Marshall, M. (2001a) 'Care settings and the care environment.' In C. Cantley (ed) *A Handbook of Dementia Care.* Buckingham: Open University Press.

Marshall, M. (2001b) 'Palliative care needs for all – responding to need not diagnosis.' *Report of a Conference of the Scottish Partnership for Palliative Care*, 21 November. Stirling: Dementia Services Development Centre.

McCarthy, M., Addington-Hall, J. and Altmann, D. (1997) 'The experience of dying with dementia: a retrospective study.' *International Journal of Geriatric Psychiatry 12*, 404–409.

McNamara, B. (2001) *Fragile Lives.* Buckingham: Open University Press.

NCHSPCS and SPAPCC (2000) *Positive Partnerships: Palliative Care for Adults with Severe Mental Health Problems.* Occasional Paper 17. London: National Council for Hospice and Specialist Palliative Care Services and Scottish Partnership Agency for Palliative and Cancer Care.

NHS Scotland (2002) *Clinical Standards: Specialist Palliative Care – Report by Clinical Standards Board for Scotland.* Edinburgh: NHS Scotland.

Oliver, M. (1996) *Understanding Disability: From Theory to Practice.* Basingstoke: Macmillan.

Sweeting, H. (1997) 'Dying and dementia.' In S. Cox, M. Gilhooly and I. McLennan (eds) *Dying and Dementia.* Stirling: Dementia Services Development Centre.

Watchman, K. (2003) *Keep Talking about Dementia.* Edinburgh: Down's Syndrome Scotland.

Wilkinson, H. and Janicki, M.P. (2002) 'The Edinburgh Principles with accompanying guidelines and recommendations.' *Journal of Intellectual Disability Research 46,* 279–284.

Woods, R.T. (1989) *Alzheimer's Disease: Coping with a Living Death.* London: Souvenir Press.

World Health Organisation (1990) *Expert Committee Cancer Pain Relief – Palliative Care. Technical Report Series No. 804.* Geneva: World Health Organisation.

CHAPTER 6

Sexuality and Dementia: Beyond the Pale?

Carole Archibald

Introduction

In this chapter I explore the subject of sexuality with specific reference to how care workers respond to expressions of sexuality by people with dementia in residential care homes. The literature points to sexuality and dementia being of concern to practitioners but marginalised in terms of research and, in practice, marginalised in discussion and training for staff. I explore some of the relevant literature and discuss some of the findings from empirical work undertaken as part of my doctoral thesis. I was interested in examining how the label of dementia influenced staff responses, and whether or not this diagnosis would further compound the prevalence of ageism, sexism and marginalisation reported in the literature in relation to sexual expression and older people.

The chapter begins with a review of the literature followed by a discussion of some of the empirical findings. The conclusions drawn are that the impact of dementia on staff responses is ambiguous and dependent on a number of factors including whether the person with dementia is seen as responsible for their actions, and the gender of the person with dementia.

The tensions and paradoxes within the literature

To provide some kind of context for the reasons the subject of sexuality and dementia has been so marginalised, there is a need to explore not only the different constructs of dementia but also those of sexuality. The complexities and tensions begin to emerge when looking at how sex/sexuality is defined in the literature.

While the focus of this chapter is that of sexuality and dementia it is important to note briefly that the marginalisation process occurs also with regard to older people and sexuality. When reviewing the literature on sexuality and older people there are gaps apparent, with the themes of neglect, ageism, homophobia and gender pertinent here also (see Archibald and Baikie 1998 for further discussion).

Defining and talking about sex/sexuality

The literal definition of sex is that it is what one does with one's genitals, with sexuality, with sometimes an ascribed identity defined through such aspects as dress and mannerisms (Hawkes 1996). Others take a more fluid approach and suggest that shifts in the meaning of sexuality have occurred over time (Caplan 1987). Sexual behaviour, practice and morality, for example, have been, and are, in a constant state of flux with strong emotional undercurrents associated with the subject.

The strong and powerful emotions mentioned above are pertinent and appear to contribute to the contradictory nature and feelings associated with the subject (Hawkes 1996). These emotions are implicated in some of the seemingly dichotomous ideas we hold about sex – pleasure and fear, control and abandon, and freedom and restriction. According to Hawkes, sexuality is mysterious, contradictory and ambiguous. It is at once private and yet public and it is teeming with inconsistencies, tensions and conflicts. In short it is difficult to define.

Ruth (1987) speaks of the dualism of two opposed realities which function to manage society's relationship to sex. To the fore are nice people behaving nicely in an antiseptic realm of non-sexuality and non-sex. Here the person is modest, covered, in control and unbothered by fantasy and dark confusions – a fantasy world itself. In the backstage area is a shameful, sin(ister), troublesome area in which dwell pleasure, pain, intensity of feeling and 'experience of carnality' (p.155) in its widest sense. These two incompatible but simultaneously operative realms of consciousness, Ruth argues, have to be balanced precariously with people learning early in life the 'intricacies of the dance' (pp.151–4).

Defining sex/sexuality is complex but there are also tensions around the vocabulary used to discuss sex. If people have difficulty in talking about sex then this may be a reason for marginalising the subject. Lawler (1991) argues that the language used about sexuality shares a similar space to the privatised body in that it is hidden away and talked of in sanitised, or vulgar, words. The biological terminology – penis, vagina, sexual intercourse – is sanitised. Historically, the slang used is frequently masculine, single-mindedly genital and was previously almost exclusively heterosexual (Ruth 1987, p.151).

The marginalisation of sexuality (and dementia) in the research process: professional danger

One possible reason for the marginalisation of sexuality as a research topic is the impact that the subject may have on the researcher's career. This is what Lee-Treweek and Linkogle (2000, pp.20–3) refer to as professional danger. These authors argue that researching sensitive subjects threatens academic conventions and may compromise the careers of researchers. Organisational research funding tends to exclude support for research topics that may be considered sensitive or detrimental to organisational interests (Troiden 1987).

Troiden (1987), in discussing research into sexuality and using Goffman's (1978) work on stigma, suggests that researchers are in some way marked when working in the field of sexuality. Others reinforce this view that researchers, in the research process, become somehow sexually suspect and personally stigmatised (Seiber and Stanley 1988). Troiden (1987), accessing the literature, notes that researchers in the area of sexuality are viewed as psychologically disturbed and can be considered either over- or under-sexed. Younger unmarried women researchers appeared to be more stigmatised than male researchers or older women researchers. The subject area is seen as somehow immoral or unnatural and by extension the researcher becomes similarly tainted. This may constrain what social scientists feel able to study in terms of obtaining funding and also with regard to the impact such research may have on their careers (Lee and Renzetti 1990).

How the constructions of dementia are part of the marginalisation process

If any discussion is to take place about the marginalisation of sexuality and dementia then an exploration of how dementia is constructed needs to be addressed. Neglect emerges as a key theme, with little theorising of dementia apparent until recently. Any conceptualising mainly occurs within the social constructionist perspective (Kitwood 1997). The theoretical gaps are arguably consistent with the power relations and the lack of influence associated with people with dementia (Harding and Palfrey 1997). People with dementia have not been 'seen' as a group as significant until recently by sociologists. In place of theory there has been a considerable body of folklore and an abundance of tacit knowledge. The person with dementia has been primarily a body with physical care needs (Kitwood and Bredin 1992). The dominant metaphor of biomedicine, the body as a biochemical machine, has predominated in the discussions.

Biomedicine and sexual expression

In the literature sexual expression by people with dementia has been largely pathologised and seen within the medical construct as challenging behaviour (Alexopoulos 1994; Cooper 1987; Haddad and Benbow 1993a, 1993b). In the medical construction of dementia, the illness has become institutionalised in the American Psychiatric Association *Diagnostic and Statistical Manual* (1980) – the DSM classification system. Dementia has become defined as a result of specific disease processes (Archibald 2003; Archibald and Baikie 1998). The biomedicalisation of both ageing and, specifically, dementia has resulted in the illness being viewed as a process of inevitable decline and irreversible decay (McColgan, Valentine and Downs 2000).

There are some apparent advantages in the certainties of the medical label of dementia. The label can legitimate an individual's bizarre behaviour and absolve him or her of responsibility for their actions (Bond 1992). However, there are also disadvantages in terms of the control exerted on the sexual expression of people with dementia, particularly when they live in residential care homes. Social control is an important part of medicalisation first conceptualised by Parsons (1951).

The part that people with dementia appear to play in this biomedical model is that of the 'sick role' conceptualised by Parsons (1951) with the resultant social control that ensues. Here the person is seen as vulnerable and thus in need of protection and/or treatment. Ethical issues are to the fore but there are difficulties apparent for the person with dementia. While there is an acknowledgement of their vulnerabilities, their competencies are often underestimated (Post 1995).

The person-centred paradigm and sexuality: a critique

Kitwood (1997) and Kitwood and Bredin (1993) have been central in the United Kingdom in offering an alternative paradigm to the dominance of biomedicine. Kitwood's work on person-centred care where the self is retrieved allows for the construction of dementia as a disability. The person here is seen as unique and valued as an individual. Their biography, their health status, their previous response to stress and their personality are all factors that will influence how they respond to dementia. Person-centred approaches, while contributing hugely to dementia care in general, are more complex when sexuality is introduced to the equation and need further scrutiny.

There seem to be gaps or contradictions apparent in the person-centred philosophy. If there is recognition that a person with the disability of dementia is an adult being with adult status then this adult may have sexual needs. Adult status includes an acceptance of a person as a sexual being and is symbolised by autonomy, self-determination and choice (Hockey and James 1993), aspects of a person's life that are central to the disability movement. These factors are often missing in the life of a person with dementia. But adult status should confer responsibility for one's own actions, which can be absent in people with dementia as the illness progresses. Sherman (1999) notes that these issues produce tensions and difficulties particularly for staff in long-term care situations. People with dementia are adults but may be deemed 'incompetent' in terms of decision making in the area of sexuality and so may be marginalised in the decision-making process (Archibald 2003).

Sexual expression not only involves the needs of the person with dementia but it can involve others whose needs also have to be considered – for example, the spouse or partner or care staff working in a residential home where residents with dementia make sexual demands (Archibald 1997). How all these needs can be met in a person-centred way can be complex and sometimes not possible.

The concept of malignant social psychology as a factor in the marginalisation process

Kitwood (1997) argues that people with a label of dementia may be subjected both internally and often externally to a debilitating onslaught that erodes their sense of personhood. They can be disempowered, infantilised and intimidated (Cheston and Bender 1999). If this concept of labelling and the consequent malignant social psychology that ensues is accepted, then it may influence how, for example, care workers respond to sexual expression by people with dementia in their care (Archibald 2002).

Dementia as disability and identity issues

Kitwood (1997) has argued that dementia needs to be seen for what it is, a disability. This perspective on dementia has helped, dramatically, to change the often nihilistic attitude of some staff/carers. The prevailing view frequently was that nothing could be done for the person. The disability model is useful in that it specifies what is missing/damaged and how people with dementia can be helped and the environment made user-friendlier (Cheston and Bender 1999; see also Oliver 1996). Using the concept of disability is of interest in addressing my research question of the role that dementia plays in care workers' response.

The literature suggests that while disabilities studies can, and have been able to, contribute to the debates by opening the doors to the cultural politics of dementia (Bartlett 2000) there are difficulties for many people with disabilities, including those with dementia, when sexuality becomes a component of their lives/care. Applying some of the ideas wholesale from the disabilities literature to the area of dementia can be problematic. For example, in terms of empowerment, the disability movement comprises young, articulate, physically disabled people, with older people and people with cognitive impairment not only excluded, but ignored. (See Bartlett 2000 for further discussion on empowerment, disability and dementia.)

Bartlett (2000) argues that the impact of the label of 'dementia' is not dissimilar to the experience of the person with a label of learning disabilities when sexual expression is a component. Similar to people with learning disabilities, the implicit role of services is often about the regulation of and the creation of sexual boundaries (Brown 1994). As with people with learning disabilities, it is questionable whether people with dementia are really free to express sexuality. There may be penalties incurred for people with dementia in breaking out of the roles prescribed for them. When people with learning disabilities express sexuality they heighten their visibility as opposed to increasing their chances of acceptance and integration (Brown 1994). These arguments may also apply to people with dementia in residential care.

Brown (1994) suggests that far from a homogeneous set of values, sexuality reveals a complex set of social rules. Following on from this one can theorise that people with dementia may be seen as 'breaking these rules' for their 'kind', with a double jeopardy for those who choose to be gay or lesbian. These issues have not generally been addressed in person-centred debates in dementia care. The 'person-centred' discussions, with a few exceptions (Archibald 1995, 1997, 2002, 2003; Kuhn 2002), may be seen as yet another debate that has marginalised sexuality as opposed to empowering and facilitating people in this area, as suggested by McLean (1994).

When looking at the literature on residential care, the identity of residents is often that of those who have failed various assessments and who are frail and dependent (Peace, Kellaher and Willcocks 1997). These are not characteristics associated with sexuality. Staff may, therefore, not perceive the resident as a sexual being and so the person with dementia's sexual needs may be neglected, marginalised or constructed as challenging behaviour; as a symptom of the disease process.

Some of the issues discussed in the literature have emerged in the findings from the following empirical work undertaken.

Sexuality and dementia: empirical work undertaken

The reasons for undertaking research in this area are worth some attention as they address the themes of the book – neglect and marginalisation (see Appendix 6.1 at the end of the chapter for research design and details of staff).

Development work undertaken with staff in residential settings suggested that the subject of resident sexuality was an issue for staff but was neglected both in policy and practice. Perusal of the literature showed a dearth of research in the area, as highlighted earlier. The question that arose was 'Why, given that the subject appeared to be such an issue in practice, was the area so neglected in policy, practice and research?' These issues were explored in a doctoral research programme.

Empirical findings

The areas discussed in this section are those which add to and are pertinent to the discussion of marginalisation and neglect. One finding within this neglected area was that there are aspects which appear to suffer further marginalisation and these would include resident-to-staff sexual expression and gay and lesbian sexual expression by residents (Archibald 2001, 2003). For the purpose of this chapter the construction of dementia and how this appears to impact on practice, with regard to resident sexual expression, will be discussed.

HOW DEMENTIA WAS CONSTRUCTED

In the residential home where the fieldwork was undertaken there appeared to be a common currency as to what was meant by the term 'dementia' when interviewing staff. Yet when I accessed the documents in the home there was a multiplicity of labels used to describe dementia (see Box 6.1). The subtleties and complexities of how dementia was constructed, and how this impacted on staff response to sexual expression by residents, only became apparent when this construction was explored in more depth.

Box 6.1 Empirical findings

Terms used to describe dementia in the staff documents:

- multi-infarct dementia
- Alzheimer's disease
- senile dementia
- dementia
- short-term memory loss
- some memory loss
- a little forgetful
- may have some dementia – difficult to say
- slightly forgetful
- mild memory impairment
- short-term memory loss – gets confused
- brain damage from alcohol abuse
- problems with short-term memory
- memory for recent events poor
- forgetfulness leading to repetition.

When asked about dementia, staff tended to have a more biomedical approach to the subject. The difficulties and stresses of the illness were emphasised.

Poor soul, it's a shame and you think what they were like years ago. Poor soul, she doesn't know what she is doing. (Interview with Evelyn, a care worker)

It's a shame because some of them are in the early stages of dementia. They know something is happening and they can get quite upset and call themselves 'stupid and thick' and it's a shame because it's not in their control. (Interview with Fiona, a care worker)

The pathos ('poor things') of the illness was emphasised. These remarks were typical and it is hard to ignore the impact that this image may have on a resident's sexual identity. Sexual expression by residents with dementia may be difficult to contemplate, especially when the dementia is more advanced.

> Like, dementia people, they're not always aware of the mess they're making toilet-wise you know and things like that, and that makes my work harder, you know? And their eating habits is, er a lot of them don't know…how can I say, where their mouth is hardly you know, they're spilling stuff, it's on the carpets. They dinn'ae bother me too much except those that are at the stage where they are moaning. I've got one that talks all the time, one who's jealous of the one that talks all the time, and she's trying to stop her and the other one making noises – whinnying you know, and that's all in one sitting room at dinner time… (Interview with Doris, a domestic)

This view of dementia provided by Doris is that of people further advanced in the illness where there may be less ambiguity about their dementia status. Ambiguity was a recurring theme when addressing the issue of sexuality and dementia. It was something that appeared to offer some explanation for the absence of reported sexual expression among residents with dementia.

THE THEME OF AMBIGUITY

When asked about the difference that dementia made to their responses when residents with dementia expressed sexuality, most staff were of the opinion that it made a considerable difference. Andrea and Marion's reports were representative of the staff group. If the person had dementia they reported that:

> I would tend to make allowances. I wouldn't consider him [she assumed I meant a him] then to be just 'a dirty old man'… (Interview with Andrea, a care worker)

> Somebody with dementia wouldn't know what they were doing. (Interview with Marion, a care worker)

Golander and Raz (2000) found in their study that dementia provided a 'halo effect' for some residents that because they had dementia they were not seen as responsible. This is reflected in the staff report above. The implications of this effect, however, may be that the person is infantilised and seen as asexual with their sexual needs not addressed. Sexual expression may not be constructed as such and/or not discussed with consequent omission from the report and thus policy documents. The difficulties were that sometimes it was unclear whether the person had dementia or not and this caused difficulties for staff in determining what action to take.

> Hmm, you see it where you'll get somebody who you think 'have they got dementia, have they not', like Michael. He's got a certain amount of dementia but not a lot, and you can sometimes think 'he's not got any dementia'. Another time you think 'Oh aye, he has got a wee bit'. And we have been told he has slightly – it doesn't come over a lot compared to someone else where you're very aware of it. (Interview with Beth, a care worker)

Another member of staff viewed the same resident, Michael, in a different way:

> As I say, if he [Michael] had dementia he had an excuse but he's not [suffering from dementia] so I dinn'ae find that acceptable of Michael. He knows everything he's doing. (Interview with Fiona)

The inference is that if someone has dementia then their actions cannot be construed as sexual. From this perspective, the difficulty in being able to interpret whether the sexual actions are the responsibility of the person or whether the behaviour is a result of dementia makes it difficult for staff to report it and even to discuss it among themselves. In the documentation of the home there was little reporting of resident-to-staff sexual expression although there had been at least two occurrences during my fieldwork at the home. It was only at the insistence of one of the care workers that a report was written in the incident book.

A finding that had implications for the reporting of sexual expression was that there were times when managers minimised incidents involving sexual expression, particularly resident-to-staff expression. Staff were sometimes seen as overreacting to the situation. Implicit was the notion that sexual expression by residents was seen as 'part of the job', institutionalised in work practice, particularly for (young) women care workers. Yet staff had received little training or anticipatory guidance for this aspect of work.

Both the culture of the home that minimised resident-to-staff sexual expression, and the ambiguity that occurred as to whether the behaviour exhibited was sexual or part of the dementing process, appeared to contribute to less openness and discussion of sexual issues in the home. Sexual behaviours, as a consequence, were either dismissed as child-like behaviour occurring in someone old and mentally incompetent and as such not constructed as sexual or, conversely, the behaviour was left ill-defined or viewed as challenging behaviour.

In residential care there is an ideology of home and the family that places a heavy burden on care workers to tolerate and, arguably, not to name this behaviour as sexual harassment. The acknowledgement that organisations are arenas of powerful sexual and emotional politics has only emerged fairly recently, through feminist studies of sexual harassment in organisations (Hearn and Parkin 1995; Parkin 1993). The construction of 'home' does not leave space for the discussion of sexually abusive behaviour within the 'home'.

FAMILY CARER INVOLVEMENT

The involvement of family appeared to be a major influence on how staff manage sexual situations and relationships in the home. Ethical issues about whether families should be involved if residents express sexual needs, and the risks involved for staff and the organisation, allow for some understanding as to why the subject has been marginalised in residential care.

Conclusions

Sexuality is a complex and ambiguous area with definitions and constructions differing over time. Sexuality is not an emotion-free zone. From the literature there appear to be powerful and contradictory emotions involved that are reflected in the polarised language used to talk about sexuality. In the empirical findings discussed in this chapter there seems to be some evidence to show that how staff perceive people with dementia in their care impacts on how the staff respond to the sexually expressed needs of residents. The evidence from this empirical work suggests also that there are areas even within this already marginalised topic that receive less attention and these would include resident-to-staff sexual expression. It is necessary to open the debates on person-centred approaches to care that are inclusive of people with dementia's sexual identity and needs; otherwise these debates, while purporting to embrace the whole individual, become part of the marginalisation process.

Omission is a powerful statement. (Starr and Weiner 1981)

References

Alexopoulos, P. (1994) 'Management of sexually disinhibited behaviour by a dementia patient.' *Australian Journal on Ageing 13*, 3, 119.

American Psychiatric Association (1980) *Diagnostic and Statistical Manual of Mental Disorders (ed3)*. Washington, DC: APA.

Archibald, C. (1995) 'Sexuality and sexual needs of the person with dementia.' In T. Kitwood and S. Benson (eds) *The New Culture of Dementia Care*. London: Hawker Publications.

Archibald, C. (1997) 'Sexuality and dementia.' In M. Marshall (ed) *State of the Art in Dementia Care*. London: CPA.

Archibald, C. (2001) 'Resident sexual expression and the key worker relationship.' *Practice 13*, 1, 5–12.

Archibald, C. (2002) 'Sexuality and dementia in residential care: whose responsibility?' *Sex and Marital Therapy 17*, 3, 301–309.

Archibald, C. (2003) 'The role dementia plays when sexual expression becomes a component of residential care work.' *Alzheimer Quarterly 4*, 2, 137–148.

Archibald, C. and Baikie, L. (1998) 'The sexual politics of old age.' In M. Bernard and J. Phillips (eds) *The Social Policy of Old Age*. London: CPA.

Bartlett, R. (2000) 'Dementia as a disability: can we learn from disability studies and theory?' *The Journal of Dementia Care*, Research Focus, September/October, 33–36.

Bond, J. (1992) 'The medicalization of dementia.' *Journal of Aging Studies 6*, 4, 397–403.

Brown, H. (1994) '"An ordinary sex life?": a review of the normalisation principle as it applies to the sexual options of people with learning difficulties.' *Disability and Society 9*, 2, 123–143.

Caplan, P. (1987) *The Cultural Construction of Sexuality*. London and New York: Routledge.

Cheston, R. and Bender, M. (1999) *Understanding Dementia – The Man with Worried Eyes*. London and Philadelphia: Jessica Kingsley Publishers.

Cooper, A.J. (1987) 'Medroxyprogesterone acetate (MPA) treatment of sexual acting-out in men suffering from dementia.' *Journal of Clinical Psychiatry 48*, 368–370.

Goffman, E. (1978) *Stigma: Notes on the Management of Spoiled Identity*. London: Pelican.

Golander, H. and Raz, A.E. (2000) 'The mask of dementia: images of "demented residents" in a nursing ward.' In J.F. Gubrium and J.A. Holstein (eds) *Aging and Everyday Life*. Massachusetts and Oxford: Blackwell Publishers.

Haddad, P. and Benbow, S. (1993a) 'Sexual problems associated with dementia: part 1. Problems and their consequences.' *International Journal of Geriatric Psychiatry 8*, 547–551.

Haddad, P. and Benbow, S. (1993b) 'Sexual problems associated with dementia: part 2. Aetiology, assessment and treatment.' *International Journal of Geriatric Psychiatry 8*, 631–637.

Harding, N. and Palfrey, C. (1997) *The Social Construction of Dementia*. London: Jessica Kingsley Publishers.

Hawkes, G. (1996) *A Sociology of Sex and Sexuality*. Buckingham: Open University Press.

Hearn, J. and Parkin, W. (1987, 1995) *'Sex' at Work*. Hemel Hempstead: Prentice Hall/Harvester Wheatsheaf.

Hockey, J. and James, A. (1993) *Growing Up and Growing Old*. London: Sage.

Kitwood, T. (1997) *Dementia Reconsidered: The Person Comes First*. Buckingham: Open University Press.

Kitwood, T. and Bredin, K. (1992) 'Towards a theory of dementia care: personhood and wellbeing.' *Ageing and Society 12*, 269–287.

Kitwood, T. and Bredin, K. (1993) 'Towards a theory of dementia care: the interpersonal process.' *Ageing and Society 13*, 51–67.

Kuhn, D. (2002) 'Intimacy, sexuality and residents with dementia.' *Alzheimer Quarterly 3*, 2, 165–176.

Kuhn, D.R., Greiner, D. and Arseneau, L. (1997) 'Addressing hypersexuality in Alzheimer's Disease.' *Journal of Gerontological Nursing*, April, 44–50.

Lawler, J. (1991) *Behind the Screens: Nursing, Somology and the Problem of the Body*. Melbourne: Churchill Livingstone.

Lee, R.M. and Renzetti, C.M. (1990) 'The problem of researching sensitive topics.' *American Behavioural Scientist 33*, 5, 510–528.

Lee-Treweek, G. and Linkogle, S. (eds) (2000) *Danger in the Field*. London: Routledge.

McColgan, G., Valentine, J. and Downs, M. (2000) 'Concluding narratives of a career with dementia: accounts of Iris Murdoch at her death.' *Ageing and Society 20*, 1, 97–109.

McLean, A.M. (1994) 'What kind of love is this?' *The Sciences*, September/October, 36–39.

Oliver, M. (1996) 'Theories of disabilities in health practice and research.' *British Medical Journal 317*, 21, 1446–1449

Parkin, W. (1993) 'The public and the private: gender, sexuality and emotion.' In S. Fineman (ed) *Emotions in Organisations*. London: Sage.

Parsons, T. (1951) *The Social System*. New York: Free Press.

Peace, S., Kellaher, L. and Willcocks, D. (1997) *Re-evaluating Residential Care*. Buckingham: Open University Press.

Post, S.G. (1995) *The Moral Challenge of Alzheimer's Disease*. London and Baltimore: Johns Hopkins University Press.

Ruth, S. (1987) 'Bodies and souls/sex, sin and the senses in patriarchy: a study in applied dualism.' *Hypatia 2*, 1, 149–163.

Seiber, J.E. and Stanley, B. (1988) 'Ethical and professional dimensions of socially sensitive research.' *American Psychologist 43*, 1, 49–55.

Sherman, B. (1999) *Sex, Intimacy and Aged Care*. London: Jessica Kingsley Publishers.

Starr, B.D. and Weiner, M.B. (1981) *Report on Sex and Sexuality in the Mature Years*. London: W.H. Allen.

Troiden, R. (1987) 'Walking the line: the personal and professional risks of sex education and research teaching.' *Sociology 15*, 241–249.

Appendix 6.1

Research design

1ST PHASE

Postal survey – structured questionnaire to managers of 28 social work residential homes in one region of Scotland (see Archibald 1997 for discussion of findings).

2ND PHASE

Fieldwork in one residential home, 'Glenevis'; three month period of observations; semi-structured interviews with most of the staff in the home; participant observation; and accessed documentation (see Archibald 2001, 2002, 2003 for discussion of findings).

PART 3

Marginalised Dementia Care Issues

CHAPTER 7

Faecal Incontinence

Christian Müller-Hergl

Faecal incontinence and nocturnal delirium are the most prominent causes for institutionalisation. From a medical point of view, incontinence and dementia are related rather by coincidence than by a causal connection. But from a socio-psychological point of view, both faecal incontinence and dementia work on a hidden agenda: that of regression (i.e. inverted human development) and dependence in institutions. Both dementia and faecal incontinence revitalise themes of dependency for all parties participating and enmesh people with dementia and paid carers in power fights concerning order and cleanliness. These can be reminiscent of the power fights between parents and children. Generally speaking dementia and incontinence highlight never-challenged or questioned relations between caregivers and persons with dementia and load these relations with old, unresolved conflicts and tensions.

How does incontinence shape and structure relations between people with dementia and professional carers within institutions? How are the institutional roles of clients with dementia and these carers constructed via incontinence? The thesis is that incontinence stabilises the caring role (i.e. the control of behaviour and effects) for professionals and helps to deny the psychosocial needs of people with dementia. Similarly, incontinence reinforces the negative identity of institutionalised individuals with dementia and their demand for attention because of their (excess) disabilities. Both roles/identities collude, presuppose and complement each other. What is avoided is the subjectivity of both parties and the possibility of personal encounter.

Vignette (see Gröning 1998)

I propose to illustrate the above thesis first through an example. A client with dementia fouls herself with faeces, her body, her face and her bed. She smears the faeces into the tiny ribs of the heater repeatedly. Staff have to clean the heater with tooth brushes. One day, staff clean her body, her bed and everything, but not her face, which is left smeared, deliberately.

The action is understood not as self-revelation (see Schulz von Thun 1994), but as something touching relation and contact. The hidden or unthematic meaning of this act of not cleaning the face can be found in interpreting it as the Cain-symbol: Cain ends his experience of being ashamed (e.g. God has not accepted his offerings but only those of his brother) by using force. Force and violence are ways to counteract perceived shame, e.g. instead of facing up to one's sadness I act out aggressively, thereby 'undoing' my fear, shame or sadness. Smearing with faeces is unacceptable and is perceived as a kind of power over the carer, an attack on his/her dignity. Returning the shame is a survival route for staff, a gesture of superiority, a reconstitution of one's position of power. The refusal of the person with dementia to accept asymmetry in the caring relationship and the refusal of humility are returned and sanctioned. In letting the client stay with a smeared face the worker violates her dignity just as much as she feels violated in her dignity, thereby satisfying a primitive balance model of justice. The experience had contradicted the professional's understanding of their role to be the one in control.

An adult person smearing oneself with faeces is an act of extreme strangeness and alien-ness. It seems that the person with dementia has a unique and horrifying power over the carer, since – not being able to abandon the active role – the carer needs to intervene, clean this up and needs to confront him/herself with this extreme strangeness. The carer cannot bypass it, cannot escape the active role, is forced to look into the pit. This hidden power within smearing violates the power of the caring role. The carer should be in the position to control, to grant attention, to say what is next. These perplexing feelings (to be in control and concomitantly lose control) are not reflected upon but instead become the source of agitation for the carer. Reflection would reveal to the carer the conflicts between the roles of the powerful helper and the realisation of powerlessness and weakness in the face of extreme strangeness. This would involve seeing smearing as possibly a way of self-expression; as a possible reaction to under-stimulation or neglect; as a call for help and contact; as an imposing performance (faeces as munition); as a sign of extreme deprivation and alienation; as a protest against social death; as a radical show of autonomy; or as a statement against the ordering and structuring powers around. Reflection and insight would at least open up the multivalent nature of acts like smearing and would allow carers to gain distance from the immediate, affective response of trying to save one's dignity in a malignant manner. In interpreting acts as being self-revelations of people's feelings and intentions – even if they do not know for sure which feeling/intention – the carers do not need to feel trapped in a situation in which they feel they need to protect themselves. Malignant reactions are a sign of power- and helplessness and of a lack of resources on the side of professionals.

Institutional matrix of action

Since incontinence is 'unacceptable' it has to disappear. The logic of exclusion gives birth to institutions, which – on behalf of the public – contain what or who is unacceptable and rejected (Gröning 2000). This in turn explains why cleanliness and order are the main focus of interest of both inspectors and the public: because these are the reasons those institutions exist.

People working there have the role of civilising and normalising, i.e. to symbolically 'undo' the alien by controlling the body, affect and behaviour. The logic of exclusion is repeated from the inside out via routines, various plans, and by defensive styles in communication and interaction which help to keep the clientele at bay (Koch-Straube 1997). Professional carers change nature into culture and contain the chaotic, the amazing and the horrible mystery of the destruction of the body and self that is caused by the illness.

The struggle for order and control is highlighted by faecal incontinence. Incontinence is often at the beginning of objectification, labelling and stigmatisation. It reduces the person to a unit to be serviced and cleaned and, within the financial and legal restrictions, reduces the caring work to body work. Individual differences do not count since the incontinence pad makes all equal. Psychosocial needs are masked, since the clean body seems to be the precondition for any possibility of contact. Everything else is important as well, but structurally of secondary importance, e.g. singing after nursing. But singing is rare, since body work consumes all caring time, which again helps professional carers to make prioritising easy. Observations of handover time show that, if the body did not need something, 'nothing' has happened. The structure of institutions constrains the awareness of individual carers.

For many professional carers there seems to be a difficulty in combining physical care or nursing with psychosocial work (Muthesius 2000). The regular transgressions into the body space seem to make it difficult to transgress into the mental, spiritual and existential dimensions of the person as well.

Enough is enough, since – vice versa – no psychotherapist cleans the bottom of his clients, only their 'mental ones'.

Mental and physical incontinence concern carers and clients alike: the body of the client lies displayed like an open landscape to be manipulated, no corner will and may be hidden from the inspecting eye. The impetus towards publication of the body results in shame and lost dignity. Clients can develop, like babies, interest in their pads, take them off and leave them full or wet on the floor or next to the remains of their last meal. They can display their faeces, play with it, eat it, smear with it, make gifts with it – wrapped or not. On the other hand, the daily loss of personal space and the invasion of private parts as public concern are routinised into work patterns that, once habitualised, tend to desensitise staff. Thus we witness staff carrying well-filled pads passing by clients who are having their meal. There can be open talk over clients' heads about whether they have had a movement. Maybe during nursing work another client in the same room has his meal, his medications, his massage or physiotherapy. Other examples include clients transported in toilet chairs to public places and toilet doors left open while in use. All this is aggravated by the extreme lack of resources, staff, education, space and finances. And after some time working there, nobody seems to mind – neither clients nor staff.

Clients in turn realise the institutional priority of the functional. They can use their deficits at least in part excessively to demonstrate power, to enforce nursing contact and to secure their role ('I am in need of help, this is evident'). When are touches, attention and body contact given, other than within functional contexts? Both sides seem to collude in invading each other's personal space – lack of concern and interest on the carer's side is answered by forcing the carer to deal with one's faeces on the client side.

Another vignette (see Gröning 1998)

A professional carer attended a private party near her place of work and on her way home visits her ward, nicely dressed and made up. She sees there a client who behaves 'improperly', playing with her food. The carer thinks that the client is doing this deliberately, since she always seems to play with food in her presence. Then the client says to her, 'You stink of garlic.' The carer retorts, 'You stink of shit.'

The client insists on symmetry in the relation and does not subject herself – she is different from other clients. The carer has made herself up nicely and thereby contrasts starkly to her normal presence and to the presence of clients, symbolically imposing in a superior position and turning up in her ward to let other people know. The client instinctively realises what she is up to, and signals this by de-throning the carer – garlic in the older generation is not a sign of good taste but rather a sign of being a stranger, foreigner or of working-class origin. The nurse returns the shame with the same impetus, with the same level of aggression and uses faecal language as munition to hurt and soil. In the end, both have soiled each other. The nurse has not been successful with her attempt to impose and impress. Her position of power has been slighted. Maybe the power fight between the two will continue, as long as the client refrains from accepting asymmetry and humility as a condition for grace.

The expression of gratitude and humility by the care recipient to the caregiver can compensate in part for a profession which is perceived at least to some extent as sewerage work. However, gratitude refused generates similar feelings to those in a parent and in particular a mother when they do not receive the respect they feel that they deserve. Only reflection on one's subliminal expectations in the professional role can provide carers with a chance to develop an independent, relaxed attitude in professional relation. Only professional distance ritualised in, for example, supervision gives the chance to be close. In that respect, a truly person-centred ability to relate to 'dependants' (children, people with handicaps, people with dementia) is a well-developed art not to be expected naturally.

Negative identity

The functioning body as an unquestioned precondition of life is often lost in very old age and indeed with incontinence. The body as integrating carrier of all dimensions of life is reduced to its deficits. The loss of inner and outer control (no longer a light 'upstairs' and tight 'downstairs') implies that the person is no longer master in one's house (Teising 1998). There is a changing perception of the body and its functions – they need anxious observation. Bodily existence and body functions are increasingly perceived as strange and alien – not as really belonging to me, to my internalised inner body picture. That is why they come into the focus of oneself and of others: the body becomes the organiser of psychosocial development in advanced old age. The centre of self-representation is the intact body – or rather the representation of the intact body. This in turn is a precondition of object-representations and so of love, affection and external interest and orientation, i.e. accepting my body/making my peace with it (even if handicapped) is a precondition to be interested in life, in objects, relations, people.

Conversely, alienation of one's body fosters a growing split between real-self (what I find I have actually become) and idealised-self (what I think I should be and which deep down I am if others were only looking properly). The result is that libido is withdrawn from object-representations back to the humiliated, deficit, disfigured body self, which starts to have a will of its own (e.g. incontinence). Thus if I am in pain I will find it difficult to enjoy buying objects that I want to have just because they are beautiful. I will find it difficult to take interest in life other than my painful and aching body and will invest all my attention towards its 'malfunctions'. The only role left is that of the patient-client imposing with diagnoses. In other words: needing help for my body becomes the prime focus of contact. In that manner the body becomes one's last ally, because its deficits constitute the high road to contact, warmth, empathy, touch. Incontinence implies both: an exclusion of contact from others and a means to enforce contact. Toileting thus becomes the currency of intimacy: who is left on the toilet longest, who is serviced immediately? Love, sympathy, attachment begin to be channelled around nursing themes, in which toileting looms large. People and relations to people are tested out by compulsory toileting habits. Thus the new staff member will be picked out in search of an ally to get me to the toilet several times an hour. Those who do not do this are 'beasts'. Occupational or music therapists in institutions who want to do therapy often, for the first couple of weeks or months, find themselves bringing people to toilets. From here it is not far to demanding more service and help than necessary, to dispensing ever more with autonomy and self-regulation to gain contact in the unsuspicious disguises of nursing care.

This negative identity is just what functionally oriented nursing care is waiting for. Excess disabilities demonstrate enormous need and justify the dominance of the body and of functional care. The incontinent client, therefore, validates the role construct of professional caregivers. This helps to minimise the psychosocial needs of people (with or without dementia) that are rather unthematically agitated upon subconsciously in incontinence work. The role construct of physical care needs the body to be controlled, cleaned and presented in a less frightening outer presentation, thereby symbolically undoing dementia. People are to appear as they would be if they did not have dementia. That is the rule of nursing homes and professionals fulfilling their part of the public contract.

The old person with dementia in turn begins to lose interest in all things except body needs. Meal times, toileting times, bathing times and the institutional rhythms that go with these close in upon the person and constitute one's only world of experience. The old person (with dementia or not) is confirmed in his/her negative identity and experiences the small world of body needs as a world not made or constructed, but as a given, unchangeable, unchallengeable reality that one has to be satisfied with. When surveyed or interviewed most elderly people with dementia will, after some time, express their satisfaction.

Both sides therefore collude in their roles, in losing subjectivity, individuality, connectedness with themselves, others and the outside world. With this goes the possibility of personal encounter, except in rare 'pockets' of caregiving, i.e. in nightshift, the occasional good morning. Both sides agree in reframing the logic of what happens here as the necessary, the pragmatic, the quasi-technical, in particular with regard to issues like incontinence. The subtext is to be pragmatic and not to talk about it. This makes it easier for both sides to conform to the rules of their role patterns.

Final vignette (see Gröning 1998)

The client, living in a religiously oriented home, cherishes and hides her faeces like a treasure to behold. It smells awfully and the carers are concerned, since the 'source' of the smell cannot be found. One day, the client is observed playing with her faeces, saying in an odd voice 'Another meatball for our Lord Jesus Christ', thereby carefully smearing the faeces into the pages of an old Bible, which in turn she puts into an old Bible box that she had brought with her when entering the institution. Carers are taken aback and take the Bible away. They are stunned and speechless, disgusted beyond words.

Public faeces separate an adult person from other grown-up humanity. A combination of faeces, sexuality and spirituality takes you ever further away – a radical antithesis to the picture of a humble, asexual, Bible-reading old woman. As usual there is an ambivalence in this act oscillating between liberation (in particular within the context of having had a religious life and living in a religious home), expression of hospitalisation, and regression to one's body and its excrements as the only source of autoerotic satisfaction. On the other, carers' side, I believe that the 'Triebangst', i.e. the angst that one has of one's basic urges and desires especially concerning sexual desire and anal regression/expression, which predominates in the 'white culture' of nurses, plays an important role in the described scene. The possibility of massive regression to basic desires and elementary modes of expressions is not a public, adult option and cannot be accepted as a life's option; on the other hand one is fascinated with this possibility, even if only in the modus of shock and denial. The logic of splitting off our own, but subconsciously suppressed, aggressive and sexual impulses, which are then magically 'worked' upon projectively in others via routines of control, cleanliness and civilised appearance, is a well-known topic within psychodynamic descriptions of professional care (Wolber 1998).

The fear of the staff who are involved with this is shown in the modes of silent, but determined, reactive aggression. This can be seen as a defence of the borders of oneself: otherwise there is no way to integrate Bible, faeces and Jesus. Possibly this reactive aggression in turn mirrors the inner reality of the client, who may be seen as absorbed by institution, old age, malfunctioning body, and by the return of destiny-like dependence on others. Maybe using religious material is contextually effective in 'unmasking' the institutional power behind the apparently loving role pattern.

Both clients and carers are inhabitants of the institution, mirroring each other, colluding with each other, buttressing each other's role, together building up institutionalised feelings (like shame, being lost, being helpless) which inform and shape the undercurrent logic of professional dementia care much more than any rational plan, management scheme, mission statement or other ideological self-descriptions. On the one hand are people fighting desperately with the remains of their identity and their new roles within the institution, on the other hand the people who have to endure this situation afresh each day. Both are there in the position of voluntary prisoners. Both may theoretically have (had) other options, but in the moment find themselves locked: although you wanted it, it turns out to be much worse than you surmised and now you cannot change it. Neither wants this situation but both are irredeemably caught up in it, since many carers have often, for a multitude of reasons, little other professional options in the moment (e.g. migrant situation). Both repeat, Sisyphus-like, the same dependency pattern every day (e.g. attachment with defence on the one hand – being essentially dependent on others like a child and resisting it at the same time – and adoption with defence on the other – being willing, and lovingly so, to accept a parent position and at the same time denying myself by returning to a controlling and regimenting parent position). Both begin to accept this as their unchangeable reality.

Body contact

Parents win power fights with very young children by giving in, securing space, letting them have their ways in defined areas and letting them explore and enjoy: their body parts, body fluids and excrements, their lust to smear and to soil, thereby losing or letting go of control in a controlled manner. This invokes the following parallel for dementia care: do not organise the day according to strict toileting patterns; do not give toileting themes great prominence and importance; try to lower the standard of hygiene, cleanliness and order. Institutions can also strengthen the psychosocial abilities and responsibilities of staff and practise the principle of least restrictive environment. They could also take care to have a skill mix in professions which does prevent the dominance of physical nursing and to have a double leadership in wards (one from the nursing section, one from the occupational/therapeutic sector) and reduce the organisational dominance of nursing in dementia care. All members of staff are responsible for nursing and occupational issues with the implication that others apart from the nursing professions do nursing jobs as well.

Most importantly, the contact points between carer and cared for need reframing and refocusing. What is needed is a function-free affective body contact independently and separately from nursing activities. Healing touches, Snoezelen, Tellington Touches (Maciejewski 2002), sensory stimulation and kinaesthetic competence come to mind in an attempt to explore access routes other than therapeutic or occupational methods. The goal in nursing becomes then to beautify rather than to clean, to continue contact and caring rather than achieving a clean and orderly state. A positive body feeling (including wellness issues) confers acceptance, security and recognition independently of toileting issues. This should happen not as something extra or by somebody 'extra' but within and integrated into the daily flow of activities. Body care is not something to get done with, but an opportunity to confer positive affect to the body.

Faecal incontinence demands a body and body-touch competence different from good functional nursing care, some of which will not be gained other than by the personal body-therapeutic experiences of carers. We are just beginning to learn how to enrich one's skills in touch, contact and being with the other person without having any nursing issue necessarily connected to this.

Nursing people with dementia needs to be seen as being essentially a therapeutic activity. This implies processes of learning which involve the carer in his/her own resources as a person. This implies to some extent the readiness to be involved in therapeutic processes over and above the job construct. A purely 'pragmatic' approach to incontinence and dementia care will miss the essential challenge within the subject of incontinence: how to build and sustain relations.

References

Gröning, K. (1998) *Entweihung und Scham. Grenzsituationen in der Pflege alter Menschen.* Frankfurt: Mabuse Verlag.

Gröning, K. and A. Abt-Zegelin (2000) 'Institutionelle Mindestanforderungen bei der Pflege von Dementen.' In P. Tackenberg and A. Abt-Zegelin (eds) *Demenz und Pflege.* Frankfurt: Mabuse Verlag.

Koch-Straube, U. (1997) *Fremde Welt Pflegeheim. Eine Ethnologische Studie.* Bern: Hans Huber Verlag.

Maciejewski, B. (2002) *KDA-Qualitätshandbuch Leben mit Demenz.* Köln: Kuratorium Deutsche Altershilfe.

Muthesius, D. (2000) 'Musiktherapie in der stationären Altenpflege.' In *Dr. med. Mabuse 25,* 127.

Schulz von Thun, F. (1994) *Miteinander Reden 1: Störungen und Klärungen.* Reinbeck: Rowohlt Taschenbuch Verlag.

Teising, M. (ed) (1998) *Altern: Äußere Realität, innere Wirklichkeiten.* Opladen/Wiesbaden: Westdeutscher Verlag.

Wolber, E. (1998) 'Von der ritualisierten Distanz in Pflegepraxis und Pflegetheorie zu einer Begegnung auf Augenhöhe.' *Pflege 11,* 3.

CHAPTER 8

Social Exclusion (and Inclusion) in Care Homes

Errollyn Bruce

Introduction

In this chapter I briefly discuss the relationship between social exclusion and institutional care, and consider the particular vulnerability of people with dementia to social exclusion. I will then use case material from a longitudinal study of well-being in residential care to illustrate three common routes to social exclusion observed among study participants.

Social exclusion and institutional care

The popular perception of care homes is not positive. For many people long-term care institutions are symbols of social exclusion, and have associations with the workhouse and memories of grim institutions encountered earlier in life. Many older people dread being 'put away' and families often carry on caring for older relatives in the face of enormous difficulties in an attempt to avoid placement in a home. Mid-20th century academic debates raised serious questions about institutional care with Goffman's (1961) powerful analysis of the devastating effects of total institutions, and Townsend's (1962) exposure of residential homes as places where independence and individuality were systematically undermined.

Although the harsh conditions of the workhouse have now gone, and the austere surroundings and rigid routines in homes and hospitals have softened, anxieties about care homes remain. These are reasonable concerns, as going into care can erode autonomy and independence, and may also put identity, dignity, intimate relationship and meaningful involvement in the wider community at risk (Peace, Kellaher and Willcocks 1997). There is recent evidence of impoverished lives and social exclusion among people in long-term care despite improved décor and mission statements about dignity and quality of life (Casey and Holmes 1995; National Institute for Social Work 1997; Royal Commission on Long Term Care 1999).

There is little doubt that institutions have a powerful potential to undermine the well-being of those who live in them but, as Gavilan (1992) noted, similar issues of dependency and control arise for frail and housebound people living at home supported by community services. Anyone needing more than ordinary amounts of help is at risk of losing power and social position. While institutional life can clearly magnify these losses, Baldwin, Harris and Kelly (1993) questioned whether this is an inevitable consequence of institutional care and Dalley (1988) argued that a long history of oppressive institutions does not mean that all forms of communal care are unacceptable. In some homes there are residents who see the move into long-term care as a positive choice and a satisfactory alternative to feeling vulnerable at home (Kellaher 2000), evidence to suggest that institutional care can be acceptable.

Despite efforts to avoid the need for institutional care, it appears to be inevitable for some people. This means that there is a need to take steps to minimise its adverse consequences and to ensure that positive experiences of life in care are not confined to a few exceptional homes (Kane 2001). Recent social policy for older people stresses the need for empowerment and inclusion (Nolan, Davies and Grant 2001). However, broad aims such as these typically take second place to keeping costs down and other pressing practical and political objectives (Harper 2000; Walker 1994). Reviewing the current literature on services for older people, Nolan et al. (2001) point out that despite many decades of commitment to laudable aims, studies on both sides of the Atlantic show that services are fragmented and patchy, with pockets of good practice and occasional shocking examples of neglect and incompetence occurring among a great deal of barely adequate provision.

The particular vulnerability of people with dementia

The pitfalls for older people in general are magnified in the case of people for whom the stigma of mental illness is added to ageing. Dementia – with its tendency to attract a malignant social psychology whereby people are depersonalised and diminished (Kitwood 1997) – brings with it additional risks of marginalisation, both inside and outside long-term care settings.

For people with dementia, institutionalisation has been, and remains, a common care solution. Recent figures suggest that around 75 per cent of the care home population has some degree of dementia, evidence that for many people with failing mental powers, institutional care is still seen as the most viable option (Macdonald *et al.* 2002). There are good reasons for this, one being the cost and difficulty of providing at home the round-the-clock support which is commonly judged to be necessary for many people with dementia at some point in their illness. Most people with dementia experience some time in institutional care, though they usually spend the majority of their time living in the community.

Active measures are needed to avert the risk of social exclusion for people with dementia wherever they live but there is particular urgency for them in long-term care settings, given the discontinuities inherent in the move into institutional care. These measures involve identifying emotional, social, occupational and spiritual needs and finding creative ways to meet them. Given the disabilities caused by dementia, this requires a special kind of care (Bruce, Surr and Tibbs 2002) based on approaches such as person-centred care (Kitwood and Bredin 1992), the person-focused approach (Cheston and Bender 1999), individualised care (Rader 1995), integrity promoting care (Brane *et al.* 1989) and the relationship approach (Zgola 1999). Many factors conspire to make this kind of care hard to achieve and maintain (Packer 2000). However, given that life for many people with dementia in care homes is highly impoverished (Ballard *et al.* 2001), small improvements can make a significant difference to well-being and quality of life.

Three routes to social exclusion in long-term care

In the remainder of this chapter I will use case material to illustrate three common routes to social exclusion and also briefly mention processes that promote experiences of inclusion. This material is taken from data collected about the lives of 93 residents with dementia who participated in a longitudinal study of well-being in residential care which took place in homes provided by Methodist Homes for the Aged,[1] an organisation with a commitment to providing care acceptable to older people, guided by holistic principles. In the course of the study we saw examples of various factors that can contribute to social exclusion, but also observed that there were many features of the care environment in these homes that enabled people to retain a meaningful sense of inclusion despite their dementia.

The three routes to social exclusion we will discuss are:

1.   The tendency for people with severe impairment and complex needs to receive little care for needs other than basic physical ones, which we refer to as an inverse care law.[2]

2.   Unfortunate outcomes of group living, bringing experiences of isolation and rejection to certain residents.

3.   Consequences of staff seeking professional advice about residents' troubling behaviour which can lead to literal exclusion in the form of admission to an assessment ward or transfer to an EMI (Elderly Mental Infirm) nursing home.

An inverse care law

The tendency towards an inverse care law has been reported by other authors (Barnett 2000; Brooker *et al.* 1998). What has been observed is that as dementia becomes more severe, the likelihood of appropriate care for emotional, physical, occupational, spiritual and social needs decreases. The reasons are relatively simple. Most staff feel out of their depth when caring for very severely impaired people. Typically they lack special skills for communicating with them and are pessimistic about the possibility that anything they do will make a difference to them. These factors are exacerbated when people with severe dementia are unresponsive and staff have no positive feedback for their efforts.

Some people with severe impairment in our study escaped the inverse care law for a variety of reasons. For example, Arnold Greenwood had qualities which facilitated responses that met his broader needs. He was active, good natured and non-threatening to staff and other residents; his non-verbal communication was good and his apparent preference for brief superficial encounters meant that he seemed content with less input than many other residents. Although very severely impaired and with little language, he had had considerably more speech when first admitted and staff used their prior knowledge of him to facilitate communication. For instance, staff would tell the jokes Arnold had told himself before his speech deteriorated, and were often rewarded with a smile.

By contrast Jean David was a classic example of someone to whom the inverse care law applied. There were many staff comments illustrating a sense of frustration with Jean:

> She worries people; you feel as if you are getting nowhere; she gets staff wound up because it feels as though she could do things but won't; she won't speak from stubbornness.

Jean responded to almost everything with what was described as *an inane grin*; the exception was personal care which she often resisted physically, and occasionally with clear sentences of protest. For the majority of the study period, opinion leaders among staff had an unsympathetic view of Jean. For example, her *bad behaviour* was blamed for an accident during an episode of personal care in which she broke her pelvis, and the possibility that this injury might cause her considerable pain was dismissed. A quiet minority dissented from the majority view, treated her with gentleness in private and claimed to have fewer problems with lack of co-operation than their less sympathetic colleagues. Jean's physical needs were attended to conscientiously, but no-one gave Jean much attention in the public areas of the home. The dominant view was that it was a waste of effort to spend time attempting to communicate with her or providing stimulation because nothing made any difference to her. The following comment, reconstructed from field notes, sums up this view:

> If you've got a bit of time to spend with someone, you wouldn't generally go to Jean David. With Jean you can't tell if anything you do makes any difference to her, she just sits there and grins whatever you do. You don't feel as though there is anything behind it. And you get the feeling that she could talk to you, but she won't, which is frustrating. All the time there's Ena, Ivy, Emily or Rose longing for a moment of your time and with any of them you can see that giving them a bit of attention makes a big difference. Apart from what has to be done for all of them, you do tend to concentrate your time where you can see it makes a difference.

'What has to be done', in this context, is physical care. Responding to other needs, though stressed in this provider's policy, was still largely seen as an optional extra by frontline staff – something also reported in other settings (Downs *et al.* 1999).

Staff said that they had to develop a view of what the people they care for are like – *how they tick* – in order to guide the manner in which they give care. Opinion leaders among staff tended to set up a dominant view of a person and their needs, and a collective 'mental set' was created with the result that staff were more likely to notice things that fitted the dominant view, and overlook or explain away things that did not.

When people are very severely impaired there are great difficulties in communicating and a good deal of guesswork and interpretation is needed, a process that is open to a large degree of error. Care staff are supposedly unskilled workers who are expected to rely upon common sense to do their work. An entirely understandable common-sense interpretation of the withdrawal often associated with severe dementia – and one frequently made by both family members and staff – is that it is an indication that people have *gone beyond* the need for emotional support, stimulation and social contact. A corollary of this view is that there is no point in attempting to provide these things, a belief which seems to underpin the inverse care law. Other processes may also be entailed. For example, many of those who remain in care work do so because it is a job where they feel they can make a difference; however, feelings of frustration and helplessness may follow when this pay-off is elusive.

Brooker *et al.* (1998) found that where the tendency to overlook people with severe dementia was discussed with staff, they recognised the problem and, given appropriate backing, were able to change their practice. In our study there were severely impaired people whose needs we felt staff had the ability to meet, but there were also some who seemed unreachable. This included a small number with very high levels of ill-being and few, if any, signs of well-being who appeared to be living in a nightmare world. Attempts to comfort them were ineffective or so short-lived that staff felt that their efforts were in vain. If there are ways to reach people like this, they go way beyond common sense and we felt that staff needed expert help and ongoing support regarding the care of these residents.

Group living

There are risks of isolation and rejection in the dynamics of group living, whether in boarding schools, barracks or care homes. In the course of the study we encountered examples of residents experiencing exclusion as a result of the actions of the resident group and also as a consequence of negative views held by staff.

Ethel Williams[3] was a proud, abrasive, self-reliant woman who had lived as an invalid for many years due to a misdiagnosis. When she came into a mixed residential home with mild dementia she had a sharp tongue and rapidly began to feel excluded, something repeatedly expressed in conversations with her researcher:

> …they all seem to get together but they don't include me and I can't go and gate-crash, I can't just go and…I can't just go and say 'Do you mind if I come

to the party?' Or, er, that's not me at all so er, I'm all right love but it's nice to see you. I'm very pleased to see you, so.

I'm all right here but er, I don't know, I'm…people don't seem to…they seem to find a partner and er…I'm sort of odd one out. All I can do is sit here in this chair.

Staff shared residents' views of Ethel, seeing her as difficult, and finding her moods unpredictable and increasingly aggressive. Most found her unappreciative, rude and hard to get close to, and there was a tense atmosphere around her. Despite this, there were frequent attempts to re-integrate her into the resident group but none were successful. Following a critical incident in the dining room where she lost her temper, and in her own terms showed herself up shockingly, she subsequently ate all her meals alone in the lounge, and the situation became more intractable. The series of taped interviews with her researcher present a heart-rending picture of an articulate woman striving to make sense of her increasing isolation, but gradually overwhelmed by a collapse of self-esteem and morale.

As we suggested in the discussion of the inverse care law, staff inevitably form a view of what residents are like – something that we all do to organise our knowledge about other people and to give us a basis for dealing with them. The nature of this view is crucial to the kind of responses that we make. Studies of common-sense explanations of other people's behaviour show that they are often superficial and based on inappropriate use of evidence (Pennington, Gillen and Hill 1999). This applies in the care context where views of others are frequently expressed using labels that stereotype and diminish the unique and complex nature of each individual (Innes 1998) and social judgements that are constantly amended and reconstructed by the staff group (Johnson and Webb 1995).

Johnson's findings from participant observation in a hospital ward resonate with our own observations. Like us, he found that a dominant ward view of patients developed in which the social judgements of opinion leaders in the staff group were influential. There were staff who felt guilty about the social judgements and labels, and some who covertly disagreed but felt unable to make an open challenge to the dominant view. Many felt that the ward view should not affect quality of care but admitted that it did. Previous work on unpopular patients had linked social judgements to patient characteristics (Stockwell 1972), but like us, Johnson found that they are constantly amended and arise from complex social processes in which staff feelings play a big part (Johnson and Webb 1995).

The staff view of Ethel was of a difficult woman, excluded from the resident group by her own rigidity and anxieties about her social position. This view was supported by the experience of their inability to find ways to intervene that enabled Ethel to negotiate a more satisfactory place in the resident group.

There were other examples where the experiences of social exclusion resulted more from staff negativity than rejection by other residents. This was clearly the case for Jean David, but also affected residents who were more mildly impaired. A complex mix of class conflict and troubling behaviour arising from deep distress led to a negative staff view of Esme Devonshire. Throughout her life, she had lived in large houses with servants. When admitted to residential care she was feeling angry and rejected by her family, and appalled by her predicament. She was not easy to deal with, being prone to angry outbursts, and physically aggressive towards staff and other residents. Although staff looked after her as well as they could, and her aggressive behaviour had improved over the time she had been in the home, they freely admitted that they resented being mistaken for servants.

During dementia care mapping, frequent allusions to her privileged background and a more authoritarian approach to her than to other residents were observed. A number of stigmatising personal detractions were recorded; for example: 'You wouldn't have used one of these [darning mushroom] because the slaves did all the work in your house.' She was not impervious to the staff view of her, and made overtures to likely visitors, particularly those with class backgrounds nearer to her own, apparently seeking acceptance and approval. Following feedback to staff the stigmatising remarks stopped, and over time the dominant view of Esme changed to a more tolerant one.

The dominant staff view of a resident seems to be a powerful factor in his or her sense of inclusion or exclusion within the home. Frontline care staff are faced with testing social situations in the course of their work, and it is not surprising that strong feelings arise following physical attacks, faecal smearing, inappropriate sexual advances, unfair accusations or cutting remarks. If there is no time to air these feelings and no safe forum in which they can be discussed, it seems inevitable that they will bias social judgements and leave residents at risk of being viewed unsympathetically. Despite attempts to be professional, unsympathetic views inevitably colour the manner in which care is given. In homes without openness to ideas and commitment to holistic care, there may be few factors acting to change negative social judgements.

Professional intervention following troubling behaviour

Among the residents in our study, those whose behaviour led to a request for professional advice faced the risk of a more literal form of exclusion – that is, transfer to another setting. For the most part only three remedies were offered in response to staff queries about behaviour they found troubling: sedative medication, admission to assessment ward or transfer to EMI nursing home. This reflects observations made by Macdonald and Dening (2002) that although 75 per cent of people with dementia in care homes have some degree of dementia, it is only if their behaviour is seen as problematic to others that specialist EMI care is considered necessary. The traditional focus of EMI care has been to control difficult behaviour rather than respond to the feelings of distress and unmet need that lie behind it. Helping people with dementia – both with and without troubling behaviour – to adjust to strange experiences of dementia and to maintain well-being despite their difficulties has not been the main focus of specialist EMI care.

Among residents in our study, sedative medication was the most common remedy offered for troubling behaviour, but in some instances admission to an assessment ward was considered, though bed shortages tended to limit this option to extreme situations. A number of residents in the study were transferred to nursing homes but intense physical care needs were as common a reason for transfer as problematic behaviour.

In the case of Maria Taylor, both medication changes and transfer were suggested. Maria was a childless widow in her early 90s who had few living relatives or friends. Although well settled in her home, she had never entirely accepted living there. Despite having moderate dementia, she was articulate and frequently talked of living elsewhere 'somewhere...near people I love' – this was impossible as all her close family were dead – and said 'it's...not like being with the loved ones that want the best things for you'. After two and a half years in the home she had a marked mental decline: staff reported increased confusion, and cognitive tests done for the study showed a substantial drop in scores. Staff began to find her aggressive outbursts harder to handle, and the dominant view was that these had become more frequent – though this was not supported by a count of entries in the daily records.

Advice was sought from the psychogeriatric service and various alterations to the anti-psychotic medication already prescribed were made. Shortly afterwards there was a very alarming incident in the middle of the night where Maria was reported to have 'completely lost control for several hours during the night...no amount of reassurance worked, she seemed to be hallucinating'.

Following this, a psychogeriatrician visited Maria, who responded to her with a major aggressive outburst. Apart from these two incidents, no other serious incidents of aggression were recorded. According to a note made by a member of staff the psychogeriatrician took the view that 'Maria is inappropriately placed in a residential home [she was in a specialist dementia residential care unit] and needs EMI nursing for her own safety and the safety of the other residents'. The anti-psychotic medication was increased, and the note recorded the doctor's advice. 'She said it may make her very flat but it would be better for her than injuring herself or others. She is going to contact Social Services...'

At this time, Maria expressed intense anxieties about rejection to her researcher. While interpretation is open to question, she was clearly distressed and expressed fears not mentioned in earlier conversations:

They are wicked people today...

Perhaps it's the woman, the mother, maybe she wasn't as nice as my own mother...

So you see, that's how they treat you, make you believe they are being kind but they're not...

Perhaps it was my own fault...they all look...they're all nice and friendly...

The referral process was slow, so by the time assessment was arranged it was agreed that Maria was 'much better'. Staff had adapted to her increased confusion, and the dominant staff view had changed to a more positive one.

Maria narrowly avoided exclusion from an environment where she was well settled and attached to staff. Despite her yearning for something better, these were her only remaining close relationships, and staying where staff knew her well was her best chance of being understood by those around her as she became progressively more impaired. It is to the credit of the staff involved that they were able to find their own solutions to the problems resulting from the changes in Maria. Her sudden decline appears to have been alarming both for her and for staff, who found that their usual ways of coping with her aggressive outbursts were no longer effective. In our view, what they needed at this point was expert support to help assess the situation, and find new ways to cope.

What they were offered did little to help them with the immediate situation, except the 'quick fix' of a different and higher dosage of anti-psychotic medication and the reassurance that they might eventually be relieved of responsibility for Maria's care. In line with evidence on the use of anti-psychotics in dementia (Ballard and O'Brien 1999; Hopker 1999) the medication changes did little to help – 'she's had a medication change but she's no different' – although some staff felt more confident when Maria was given stronger sedative medication.

The difficulties that staff face in coaxing highly anxious and panicky people with dementia through the daily indignities of having help with personal care and other frustrations of living with dementia should not be under-estimated. But from the residents' point of view, insult is added to injury if the solution to these difficulties is to exclude them from settings which have become familiar. Other research has shown that people with behaviour seen as challenging sometimes experience a series of transfers, a remedy that does little to tackle their underlying problems (Moniz-Cook, Millington and Silver 1997; Silver, Moniz-Cook and Wang 1998). A more effective approach is to provide ongoing specialist support for staff to help them to identify and respond to the needs underlying the troubling behaviour (Moniz-Cook 1998; Perrin and May 2000). In our view, specialist support of this kind would be more valuable to staff than the medication changes and transfers that are more commonly offered by supporting professionals.

Routes to social inclusion

It would give an unbalanced picture of the lives of the residents in our study to describe the routes to social exclusion with no mention of the dynamics of inclusion. Residents pursued a number of different strategies to gain what we came to call 'a place in the sun' within the context of communal care, and the success of these strategies was dependent to a large degree on positive attitudes and tolerance from staff. Experiences of social inclusion were achieved using a variety of different strategies such as taking up a 'top dog' position within the resident group; becoming a staff 'pet' through being affectionate, appealing and responsive; being given tender care as a result of having much to contend with and bearing it bravely; being respected as a character; making people laugh; and becoming an honorary member of the staff team. These strategies involved an interplay between residents' retained social skills and attempts to find a comfortable niche in the group and staff understanding of residents as active agents and recognition of their need to 'keep their end up despite dementia'.

The majority of residents in our study maintained moderate or high levels of well-being over a period of time, something which seemed to be the result of the interaction between their concerted attempts to cope with the disabling impact of dementia and the special atmosphere in the study homes. This was summed up by one relative as 'care that goes far beyond "legal requirements"', and a significant element in the special atmosphere was the enabling social environment arising from the assumption that behind the manifestations of dementia there are people still able to make something of their lives.

Conclusions

In all the routes to social exclusion and inclusion discussed here, staff views of residents played an important role. Negative views were associated with pessimism and detachment, driving the belief that nothing can be done to help people who are severely impaired, unpopular within the group or under threat of transfer. Positive views enabled people to find and maintain a niche within the social group, and helped to protect them from exclusion when their care needs became intense.

Given the unusual social situations that occur in the course of giving care to people with dementia, it is not surprising that staff relying on common sense tend to make negative social judgements about people in their care. Common sense typically takes a dim view of people who are unrewarding, upsetting or create unnecessary extra work, and has low expectations of those who are old and mentally impaired. The care that follows from negative social judgements often exacerbates experiences of social exclusion, and increases the chances that people remain unrewarding, upsetting and hard work to care for, thereby confirming the common-sense position. Organisational commitment and strong leadership towards positive views of people with dementia can do much to ameliorate the negativity of common-sense social judgements and to underpin a kind of care that brings rewards for hard work, and resolution of upsetting experiences. This kind of care can foster experiences of social inclusion.

In general, dementia is still predominantly understood as a devastating condition about which little can be done. Inevitably this social context limits the possibility of a special kind of care for people with dementia, as the predominant view shapes the social judgements of professionals, care staff, families and people with dementia themselves. As well as individual and organisational commitment and understanding, a much greater degree of dementia friendliness – and a realistic acceptance of ageing – is needed in society as a whole if we are to minimise the risk of social exclusion for people with dementia in long-term care.

Notes

1 Now known as MHA Care Group.

2 We borrowed the idea of an inverse care law from Tudor-Hart (1971) who used it to refer to regional inequalities in health services, having observed that in areas where needs were greatest there was the least availability of good medical care.

3 All residents' names are pseudonyms.

References

Baldwin, N., Harris, J. and Kelly, D. (1993) 'Institutionalisation: why blame the institution?' *Ageing and Society 13*, 1, 69–81.

Ballard, C. and O'Brien, J. (1999) 'Treating behavioural and psychological signs in Alzheimer's disease.' *British Medical Journal 319*, 138–139.

Ballard, C., Fossey, J., Chithramohan, R.H., Burns, A., Thompson, P., Tadros, G. and Fairbairn, A. (2001) 'Quality of care in private sector and NHS facilities for people with dementia: cross sectional survey.' *British Medical Journal 323*, 426–427.

Barnett, E. (2000) *Including the Person with Dementia in Designing and Delivering Care: 'I need to be me.'* London: Jessica Kingsley Publishers.

Brane, G., Karlsson, I., Kilgren, M. and Norberg, A. (1989) 'Integrity-promoting care of demented nursing home patients: psychological and biochemical changes.' *International Journal of Geriatric Psychiatry 4*, 165–172.

Brooker, D., Foster, N., Banner, A., Payne, M. and Jackson, L. (1998) 'The efficacy of dementia care mapping as an audit tool: report of a 3-year British MHS evaluation.' *Ageing and Mental Health 2*, 1, 60–70.

Bruce, E., Surr, C. and Tibbs, M.A. (2002) *A Special Kind of Care: Improving Well-being in People Living with Dementia.* Derby: MHA Care Group, www.methodisthomes.org.uk

Casey, M.S. and Holmes, C.A. (1995) 'The inner ache: a experiential perspective on loneliness.' *Nursing Inquiry 2*, 3, 172–179.

Cheston, R. and Bender, M. (1999) *Understanding Dementia: The Man with Worried Eyes.* London: Jessica Kingsley Publishers.

Dalley, G. (1988) *Ideologies and Caring: Rethinking Community and Collectivism.* London: Macmillan.

Downs, M., Gilloran, A., Crossan, B. and Thomas, J. (1999) *Changing the Culture of Care: The Effect of Resettlement on Staff.* Final report to the Chief Scientist Office of the Scottish Office Home and Health Department, Edinburgh.

Gavilan, H. (1992) 'Care in the community: issues of dependency and control – the similarities between institution and home.' *Generations Review 2*, 4, 9–11.

Goffman, E. (1961) *Asylums.* London: Penguin Books.

Harper, S. (2000) 'Ageing 2000: questions for the twenty-first century.' *Ageing and Society 20*, 1, 111–122.

Hopker, S. (1999) *Drug Treatments and Dementia.* London: Jessica Kingsley Publishers.

Innes, A. (1998) 'Behind labels: what makes behaviour "difficult"?' *Journal of Dementia Care* 6, 5, 22–25.

Johnson, M. and Webb, C. (1995) 'Rediscovering unpopular patients: the concept of social judgement.' *Journal of Advanced Nursing 21*, 466–475.

Kane, R.A. (2001) 'Long-term care and a good quality of life: bringing them closer together.' *The Gerontologist 41*, 3, 293–304.

Kellaher, L.A. (2000) *A Choice Well Made: 'Mutuality' as a Governing Principle in Residential Care.* London: Centre for Policy on Ageing/Methodist Homes.

Kitwood, T. (1997) *Dementia Reconsidered.* Buckingham: Open University Press.

Kitwood, T. and Bredin, K. (1992) 'Towards a theory of dementia care: personhood and well-being.' *Ageing and Society 12*, 269–287.

Macdonald, A.J.D. and Dening, T. (2002) 'Dementia is being avoided in NHS and social care.' *British Medical Journal 324*, 548.

Macdonald, A.J.D., Carpenter, G.I., Box, O., Roberts, A. and Sahu, S. (2002) 'Dementia and use of psychotropic medication in "non-EMI" nursing homes in South East England.' *Age and Ageing 31*, 1–7.

Moniz-Cook, E.D. (1998) 'Psychosocial approaches to challenging behaviour in care settings – a review.' *Journal of Dementia Care 6*, 5, 33–38.

Moniz-Cook, E.D., Millington, D. and Silver, M. (1997) 'Residential care for older people: job satisfaction and psychological health in care staff.' *Health and Social Care in the Community 5*, 2, 124–133.

National Institute for Social Work (NISW) (1997) *Measuring the Quality of Residential Care.* NISW Briefing No. 21. London: NISW.

Nolan, M., Davies, S. and Grant, G. (2001) *Working with Older People and their Families: Key Issues in Policy and Practice.* Buckingham: Open University Press.

Packer, T. (2000) 'Does person-centred care exist?' *Journal of Dementia Care*, May/June, 19–21.

Peace, S., Kellaher, L. and Willcocks, D. (1997) *Re-evaluating Residential Care.* Buckingham: Open University Press.

Pennington, D.C., Gillen, K. and Hill, P. (1999) *Social Psychology.* London: Arnold.

Perrin, T. and May, H. (2000) *Well-being in Dementia: An Occupational Approach for Therapists and Carers.* London: Churchill Livingstone.

Rader, J. (1995) *Individualised Dementia Care: Creative Compassionate Approaches.* New York: Springer.

Royal Commission on Long Term Care (1999) *With Respect to Old Age.* London: HMSO.

Silver, M., Moniz-Cook, E.D. and Wang, M. (1998) 'Stress and coping with challenging behaviour in residential settings for older people.' *Mental Health Care 2*, 4, 128–131.

Stockwell, F. (1972) *The Unpopular Patient.* Beckenham, Kent: Croom Helm.

Townsend, P. (1962) *The Last Refuge: A Survey of Residential Institutions and Homes for the Aged in England and Wales.* London: Routledge and Kegan Paul.

Tudor-Hart, J. (1971) 'The inverse care law.' *The Lancet,* 27 February, 405–412.

Walker, A. (1994) *Half a Century of Promises.* London: Counsel and Care.

Zgola, J.M. (1999) *Care That Works: A Relationship Approach to Persons with Dementia.* London: Johns Hopkins Press.

CHAPTER 9

Risk Taking

Jill Manthorpe

Unlike many of the subjects covered in this book, risk is not one that has only recently attracted attention. Risk permeates discussion of dementia and causes concern, anxiety and indecision. In this chapter, the focus is on risk taking, largely within professional practice. It starts with a brief discussion of risk and some of the themes that have emerged in debates about risk in dementia support. It then offers some points for positive risk taking set in the context of services in the community and residential settings.

Thinking about risk and dementia highlights two features of current conceptualisations of risk. The first reminds us that risk within mental health services and policy is regarded with caution, if not anxiety. The second construct is that social acceptance of risk taking is becoming synonymous with adult status (while children are deemed to need increasing levels of surveillance and protection). The status of older people, however, is sometimes seen as less than fully adult. Risk taking in dementia is therefore influenced by debates that take place outside the dementia arena, those about the contentious areas of mental health and those in the ambiguities of ageing.

Dementia often gives rise to difficulties in functioning, in memory and in dealing with the risks of ordinary life (though these are not confined to dementia). It is rare that we consider how risk is managed when such difficulties arise: how people hold on to their previous skills in negotiating ordinary risky environments and relationships. Instead we focus on danger. This leads to technical aspects of risk infiltrating ordinary life: we are all to become experts in risk assessment, we all need educating about risk factors and we all have to become risk decision makers in the fields of personal finance, healthcare and social relationships. Whether or not we see risk as a matter of balancing possible gains with possible disadvantages, the role of the individual is to make a rational calculation.

For people with dementia, risk taking in the past may be forgotten and previous attitudes or patterns of behaviour may be shifting. A person with dementia, for example, may now be seeking security or appear to welcome routine, in contrast to earlier characteristics. While enhancing risk may figure in discussions about problems when supporting people with dementia, it is important to listen to experiences that illustrate that some people with dementia appear risk averse and are fearful at times. This is evident from reports of carers about everyday life; Anne Simpson (Simpson and Simpson 1999), for example, draws on her experience to advise other carers that people with Alzheimer's may feel anxious continually:

> Most partners are deeply afraid of being abandoned: Many of them shadow their caregivers. 'Where are you? What are you doing?' They stroke and pat us to reassure themselves of our presence. (p.147)

Carers, trying to manage their own risks, may become overwhelmed by the many pulls about doing what is best for the person with dementia, for the carer themselves and for other significant family members. Much risk discussion focuses on the carer–person with disability dyad: less places either in a broader setting with multiple risk judgements and perspectives.

The professional perspective may also include elements of risk taking. It is often said that a blame culture has infiltrated health and social care, and that blame is the unjust process that promotes professional conservatism (see Alaszewski, Harrison and Manthorpe 1998). How practitioners negotiate care environments which are said to be risk averse and whether those which promote risk taking lead to the anticipated improvements in quality of life remain hypotheses. Although some indication of this might arise from a study of policies, and there are numerous versions of risk policies or similar documents, what goes on in practice may be different from written guidance (Manthorpe 2003).

Dementia care presents a range of opportunities to consider how risk permeates ordinary life. We know something of risk in relation to the 'big' issues, often where professionals predominate, such as rights and risk over restraint and medication. We know less about how home care workers and residential care staff manage risk in ordinary events and encounters, both risks faced by people with dementia and also risks from staff's own behaviour and practices. Similarly, while we know something of the world of those family carers supporting people with dementia, we know less of how they balance, strike compromises or negotiate various risks when different obligations appear to compete. And the voice of people with dementia is, as in many areas, only emerging (see Wilkinson 2002).

Thinking about and responding to risk in dementia care may profit from a focus on the small, on activities of daily life, as much as on the major dilemmas. While debates about a 'risk society' tend to look at major social movements, thinking small may help identify individual patterns, preferences and priorities. The six sections below in the main use examples of everyday decision making, though exposure to global risks, such as pollution, and economic risks, such as the transfer of health costs back to individuals and their families in the UK, impact upon people with dementia as they do upon us all.

Recognising risk

Risk may be defined as danger, or as potentially liberating or as a process of calculation of the likelihood of negative outcomes occurring. The recognition, management and assessment of risk for its citizens is a central responsibility of government. A recent Cabinet Office document outlined the UK government's desire to improve decision making and risk handling, to ensure fewer surprises and to better manage the unexpected, to enhance public confidence and understanding of risk, and to reach greater consensus about balances and trade-offs (Strategy Unit 2002). Most welfare agencies would recognise the desirability of this.

Within welfare services likewise, risk assessment and management are increasingly accepted as a key professional and service activity (Stalker 2003). The uncertainty its definitions entail seems to resonate with the difficulties of health and social care practice. For example, the point made by the white paper *Modernising Social Services* (Department of Health 1998) could apply to dementia support in particular: '…people who work in social care are called on to respond to some of the most demanding, often distressing and intractable human problems' (Department of Health 1998, 5.2, p.84).

With the development of high thresholds before entitlement to social care services and the rationing of healthcare, managing risk has replaced meeting need as a key objective. As Kemshall (2002) noted, if meeting need is replaced by managing risk as the remit of welfare then the 'nettles' of risk have to be grasped. This means that those services treading the taut wire between empowerment/protection and control have to respond to demands to recognise when risks are dangers and when the costs of action outweigh the costs of inaction. It also means that risk becomes defined as danger, an outcome that is negative and one that seems likely to present harm to service users, practitioners and conceivably the public. If defined this way then the management of risk is a one-way process of risk minimisation. One Social Services Inspectorate report, for example, illustrated that staff in recognising risk were identifying dangers:

> Managers and staff indicated that considerations of risk were to the forefront of their minds when organising and delivering services – hence their readiness to pinpoint gaps and shortcomings. (Social Services Inspectorate 1989, p.64)

This recognition of risk as danger serves to suppress definitions of risk as liberating and as part of the experience of ordinary life, particularly for adults. Some forms of risk taking constitute activities that are highly valued and enjoyed. This positive definition of risk is more likely to be found in services that have embraced a philosophy of normalisation, such as those influenced by ideas about learning disability that emphasise social inclusion or rights (Alaszewski *et al.* 2000), but elements of it are to be found in policy pronouncements about services for older adults. Paternal or maternal attitudes to them can undermine older people's confidence. It is recognition of this that led perhaps to the *National Service Framework for Older People* (Department of Health 2001, p.27) asserting:

> OLDER PEOPLE SHOULD BE INVOLVED IN MAKING THEIR OWN DECISIONS...

> It is also for the older person to determine the level of personal risk they are prepared to take when making decisions about their own health and circumstances.

How far then does that apply to people with dementia? Are they to be seen as rational risk assessors, able to balance the positive and negative elements of risk assessment or is their ability to recognise risks compromised so far that proxy risk decision makers have to take on this role? The following sections explore these questions.

Refining

One of the results of seeing risk as danger is that differences in the seriousness of the anticipated outcome and between probabilities become eclipsed. If something is labelled as a risk then there is a tendency to treat the risk as highly likely or even certain, causing anxiety as witnessed by scares over food safety, child abuse, crime and technology, to give examples from recent risk stories. In the UK, the 'mad-cow' disaster prompted the government to consider how best to make the public more risk literate. The BSE Inquiry (Phillips 2000) spent some time arguing that zero risk was not feasible but that likelihood of harm and severity of harm could be identified (p.31) and that the public should be given such information rather than reassurance (p.xviii). In other words, risk assessments should be undertaken and their results communicated.

For practitioners, risk assessments, on their own or as part of other assessments, are ways of scanning the environment for intelligence about risks, or rather hazards. This is not a role unique to welfare; as Giddens (1999) observed in his Reith lectures, risk assessment is a global industry and part of the institutionalisation of risk: 'A significant part of expert thinking and public discourse today is made up of risk profiling – analysing what is the current state of knowledge, in the distribution of risks.'

Risk assessment is as much an art as a science in that it builds on shaky and incomplete evidence bases and incorporates values and images, emotions and contexts. As Calman, Bennett and Coles have shown (1999), we are more likely to fear and overestimate risks that are vivid, invisible and affect the innocent. This may explain the concern about people with dementia causing major accidents by 'leaving the gas on', a severe outcome if an explosion occurs of course, but one which is dramatic: its build-up is invisible and insidious, and the consequence may harm 'innocent' neighbours. Understanding the fear behind such concerns may help practitioners to respond to anxieties that they think are based on gross exaggerations of risk, whether these emanate from family or fellow practitioners.

Risk assessment is part of general assessment but it may be more specialised if certain contexts apply. Returning home from hospital is one example of a complex set of risk assessments, some of them formalised. At one level, a multidisciplinary team or perhaps a single medical practitioner will consider the ability to benefit from hospital stay or treatment. The risks of going home may be assessed by a physiotherapist or occupational therapist. Discussions may be shared between the hospital team, involving relatives and the person with dementia, in theory at least, both to share understandings of risk and to consider how they will be managed.

Such processes involve the reaching of agreement about individual risks and the ways in which they will be negotiated. Living on one's own, for example, may be seen as a risk for a person with dementia and yet this is common among people with dementia, especially in its early stages. In a study of ten people with dementia living on their own, Gilmour, Gibson and Campbell (2003) identified that people who might easily be labelled as being at risk because they lived alone were sometimes able to manage risks because of factors which prevented, or were able to respond to, situations of harm. At times relatives and neighbours in this rural area were in daily contact with the person with dementia and this provided some level of monitoring. Their relationship meant that this social support was embedded in a familiar context, and that patterns of behaviours were known so that the out of the ordinary could be addressed and harm minimised. For example, a bank employee recognised that a stranger was accompanying a person with dementia to withdraw cash from the bank and alerted the family to this unusual occurrence. A risk assessment that focuses purely on the deficits of cognitive functioning would miss this potential ability of social support to enable a person with dementia to continue to live at home relatively independently. While the risks of financial abuse might be evident, their likelihood can be reduced, if never completely annihilated, unless the person with dementia is stripped of all their income and assets.

For practitioners, the message appears to be that risk should not be avoided or ignored as an example of ageism or oppression. It should instead be named and assessed. Then a process of negotiation can follow. In the next section the capacity of the person with dementia to undertake these processes will be discussed.

Considering capacity

Adams (1995, p.2) has described how adults take most decisions about risk involving young people and how there is a gradual transfer of responsibility as adulthood approaches. But he observed that a third tier of responsibility is evident, for those adults who are not considered responsible or capable of making risk decisions, and this is at the level of authorities who act as parents when adults are not deemed to be sufficiently trustworthy or well informed. People with dementia may seem a good example of those whose adult status has been superseded, but mental capacity is presumed to exist unless evidence is there to the contrary, and capacity under English law depends on a person's ability to receive and retain information, not to agree with it. In other words people do not have to act sensibly. Their capacity also relates to the importance of the decision with higher levels of understanding required for some decisions than others.

For practitioners, establishing mental and legal capacity can be a mine-field. The law in England is the result of accumulations of statute and responsibility for assessing mental capacity can be undertaken by a variety of professionals. The Law Commission (1997) has made proposals for clarifying the law in recognition that growing numbers of people with dementia mean that current uncertainties over matters such as consent, contracts, protection and risk increasingly present services and families with unnecessary trouble and distress and these look likely to be the subject of legislation. In Scotland, the Adults with Incapacity Act 2000 established a formal process of substitute decision making for people with dementia among others: it will be important to see whether this enhances quality of life. But regardless of the precise legal frameworks, what remains for authorities, to use Adams' (1995) term, is an exercise in balancing rights to self-determination with the need for protection from harm. This image of balance is commonly adopted in relation to risk for older people with mental health problems; but balance may be an inaccurate simile as changes occur fairly frequently when supporting people with dementia.

For example, a person may have understanding in some areas and not oth-ers or the level of their capacity may be fluctuating. Here practitioners may find it helpful to seek the support of others in setting out the basis for risk tak-ing or otherwise. Recording the basis of their assessments is also valuable. While there is a possibility that advance directives, setting out a person's wishes in the event of loss of capacity, may offer guidance to services about a person's preferences or choices, these are not yet commonplace. Moreover they may be very general and will need interpretation and application in the light of the dilemmas of the time. Such discussions will often involve reaching a consensus with carers and it is the perspectives of families that are explored next.

Widening the net

While risk is a professional concern it is evident that carers, those supporting people with dementia at home, also engage in the risk enterprise: they assess, manage and monitor risks. Buri and Dawson (2000) used the example of the risk of falls among people with dementia to explore how family carers viewed these risks and the strategies they developed to reduce them. They found that 'carers were constantly on patrol' (p.288), looking out for dangers and being highly sensitive to change or movement. They gathered information about previous falls about precipitating factors. In managing risks, some carers used various means of control to reduce the likelihood of a fall, such as limiting the ability of the person with dementia to move around by blocking them in with furniture. They selected advice from professionals if it seemed appropriate to their circumstances.

For practitioners the message is therefore that carers manage a range of risks and that a didactic approach, based on an objective assessment and then telling carers what to do, is unlikely to be welcome or acceptable. Buri and Dawson (2000) suggested that it is helpful to identify individual carers' understandings of risk and to help carers consider and learn from their own experiences. There is an unspoken dilemma in their acknowledgement that sometimes carers' control or use of restraint may provide carers with peace of mind, but may inhibit the independence of the person with dementia to an unacceptable degree.

Carers' understandings of risk may not always accord with those of professionals as examinations of their discussions have also indicated (Adams 2001). This observation exposes the imprecision of risk assessments, many of which have to be completed in the presence of carers as informants. If a carer wishes to avoid a subject or to present it in a certain light, then it seems that this is possible. Conversely, a risk may be identified through conversation with carers that has not previously been considered, as Adams' report of a meeting between a community psychiatric nurse (CPN) and a carer illustrated when the alcohol consumption of the person with dementia was explored by the CPN following a chance remark (Adams 2001, p.313).

Clarke and Heyman (1998) suggested that there are different knowledges of risk between professional and lay carers. A family member may have specific, individualised knowledge and experience of the person with dementia. Practitioners' knowledge is derived from training and enhanced by professional encounters and experiences, particularly instances of crisis and difficulty. While professionals' risk expertise is dominant, professionals may be more effective if their practice was more respectful of lay perspectives and, as a result, if it relied less on generalities.

Risk, however, is often assessed and managed within multidisciplinary and multi-agency settings, sometimes involving teams but otherwise involving series of overlapping conversations and written communications. It is a mistake to see risk assessments as merely those documents with such a label, for they are part of the daily discussions and correspondence of professional interaction, such as case-notes, reports, referrals and reviews. As the above sections have argued, definitions of risk may vary and it may be helpful for precision about the term to be part of professional communications, with room to observe that there is inevitably much uncertainty. While some have argued that it might be possible to construct a common clinical language around risk (Misselbrook and Armstrong 2002) to assist professionals, this misses the subjectivity and value-laden dimensions that seem to affect professionals as much as the lay public. Differences exist between professionals and between families of course, and it is to the issue of conflict that the next section turns.

Considering conflict

One of the 'high priests' of risk, sociologist Ulrich Beck, has recently been criticised for downplaying the issues of power and domination in his discussions of risk (Elliott 2002). At the level of supporting individuals with dementia, power and conflict are inherent in discussions of risk, if generally under-stated. Some associate the blandness of debate with general negative attitudes towards risk taking among older people, such as their right to take risks in respect of alcohol. Herring and Thom (1997), for example, found that services had not solved what they saw as a dilemma in balancing risks with a philosophy of rights (p.243). Among very old people, Bury and Holme (1991) found that avoidance of all risks was not always the highest priority and asked: 'The question, therefore, is how much risk for extremely old, possibly frail, people is acceptable and whose definitions of risk should prevail?' (p.130).

People with dementia may lack power and thus their perspectives on risk may be negated or ignored. It may be easy to see relatives as controlling but increasingly studies of carers show that they are conscious of the impact of their risk decisions. Parker (1993) found that spouse carers appreciated the inherent tension between their desire to protect and their partners' need for independence and risk taking. Likewise, Marian Barnes (1997) reported that the carers interviewed in her study recognised possible power differentials:

> Carers are often aware of the potential for conflict between their own needs and those of the people they support. Respite care is a good example of this. Carers need a break from caring but they know that often the person they care for does not want to be 'pushed out' into a respite care home to enable this to happen. They face the dilemma of forcing their relative to do something which will make them distressed or unhappy, or risking their own health by not taking a break. (p.110)

In other circumstances conflict may occur, when differences in values are exposed or when there are disagreements over responsibility, property or treatment. People with dementia themselves may not wish for information to be passed to their family about events which may expose their vulnerability. Clark, Dyer and Horwood (1998), for instance, gave an example of a person who did not want her neighbours to tell her family that she had fallen because of their anticipated alarmist reactions.

However, conflict or differences in perspective between people with dementia and those providing their care may be muted for other reasons. Martin and Bartlett (2003) have illustrated how people with dementia may find it very difficult to be heard when risks are being set out in a decision-making forum. In one example where professionals were deciding that a person with dementia should move into a nursing home, the person reported how she felt it had been hard to participate in the meeting, feeling ill-prepared, out-numbered and having no representative. The final section moves to consider further the perspectives of people with dementia in relation to risk taking.

Living with risk

People with dementia are often considered to have enhanced vulnerability to risk as danger and to have diminishing capacity to deal with risks rationally. This leads to a protective approach in their own best interests which is the dominant theme in discussions about professional accountability and duties of care. Such a defensive position is understandable in a litigious climate, where blame and scapegoating are feared. It is also understandable when the risks that a person with dementia wishes to undertake do not simply affect him or herself but may cause harm to others. This issue can be illustrated by the example of driving that, as more older people have access to their own cars, increasingly may be an area of conflict between those who think that the risks of continuing to drive are too great and those who wish to continue to drive.

Driving is an activity that may be valued highly but it may be an activity that a person with dementia relinquishes voluntarily. For some it is a significant activity and status that they wish to retain and they do not agree with assessments of general risk that it is not safe for them to drive any more. The feelings involved were articulated by Bob, for example, in Snyder's (1999) collection of interviews with people with dementia. Bob observed: 'Losing my driver's license was like somebody cutting off my arm. I lost something that was a part of myself. I lost my freedom primarily' (p.90).

Bob outlined how he felt this was unjust, he had never had an accident, he was not told the reason, and he felt he should have been able to appeal against the decision (p.88). In contrast, he reported how he had voluntarily given up his hobby of woodwork, in recognition of the dangers this represented. This example presents a picture of someone who is able to assess risk, by undertaking a process of calculating likelihood and outcome, but, like most of us, draws on a unique pattern of experience and feels that generalisations do not always apply to individual circumstances. Should the activities of driving and woodworking have been reversed and Bob wished to continue his woodwork hobby and not his driving, then it may be that he would have been given support and assistance to take risks which exposed him to an element of danger, but less so others. Unfortunately for Bob's point of view the risk taking he desired was in an area where there is a legal framework to protect others and their interests over-rode his own desires.

This example illustrates for practitioners that risk is context specific and that while positive risk taking may be encouraged, it is set within frameworks which see people with dementia as vulnerable and as less than capable of undertaking risk assessments and managing risks than other adults. People with dementia cannot be expected to be better risk assessors than other people, since most of us are amateurs in measuring uncertainty. Practitioners can play a key role in highlighting the contradictions between clamours for protection and safety and calls for choice and ordinary life. Dementia support is also one area where the simplistic distinction between risk assessment and risk management breaks down. People with dementia, as Bob's story illustrated, need support during assessment and in managing risks.

Conclusion

Risk then is a unifying theme in welfare and for those working in dementia support it is helpful perhaps to see that all agencies and practitioners face similar tensions. One of the outcomes of service re-organisation in the UK recently has been a growing divergence between areas such as mental health, child welfare and older people's services. An occasional flurry of interest occurs when links are recognised, such as the impact of disability across family members, but professions, practitioners and providers are increasingly specialised.

Twenty years ago Mary Marshall (1984) identified fear and ignorance as reasons for the taboo status of dementia. Fear lay behind people's unwillingness to consider this as their own possible future while fear of an upsurge in service demand from growing numbers of people with dementia and their carers was evident among professionals and policy makers. Marshall set out a range of strategies to break the taboo of dementia and to some extent these have been achieved: there is more information, greater sharing of problems and solutions, increased recognition of stress, some better (though insufficient) resources and an environment of change.

Challenges remain of course and we are learning more of the complexity of disabilities such as dementia and the ways in which people's support is undermined if it concentrates on managing risk and not meeting personal needs. A recent survey of service providers (Daker-White *et al.* 2002) demonstrated how pernicious this view might be: '...the general attitude of staff in mainstream services is that people with dementia are a problem, a risk and a security issue' (p.107).

If people with dementia are seen as personifications of risk, then there is greater likelihood that fear and ignorance will govern assessments and risk management. However, risk cannot be managed by denial: it is too ubiquitous a theme to be sidelined or swept under the carpet. Risk needs to be named and its dimensions explored through discussions with people with dementia, their carers and a range of practitioners. Conflict is inevitable as individuals will pitch the fulcrum between independence and protection in different places. Finding a language to discuss the risk in question is important but this language will need to address conflict and not assume that risk assessments are universally agreed as beneficial or person centred.

References

Adams, J. (1995) *Risk.* London: UCL Press.

Adams, T. (2001) 'The social construction of risk by community psychiatric nurses and family carers for people with dementia.' *Health, Risk and Society 5*, 3, 307–320.

Alaszewski, A., Alaszewski, H., Ayer, S. and Manthorpe, J. (2000) *Managing Risk in Community Practice: Nursing, Risk and Decision-Making.* London: Balliere Tindall.

Alaszewski, A., Harrison, L. and Manthorpe, J. (eds) (1998) *Risk Health and Welfare.* Buckingham: Open University Press.

Barnes, M. (1997) *Care, Communities and Citizens.* Harlow: Longman.

Buri, H. and Dawson, P. (2000) 'Caring for a relative with dementia: a theoretical model of coping with fall risk.' *Health, Risk and Society 2*, 3, 283–294.

Bury, M. and Holme, A. (1991) *Life After Ninety.* London: Routledge.

Calman, K.C., Bennett, P.G. and Coles, D.G. (1999) 'Risks to health: some key issues in management regulation and communication.' *Health Risk and Society 1*, 1, 293–300.

Clark, H., Dyer, S. and Horwood, J. (1998) *'That Bit of Help': The High Value of Low Level Preventable Services for Older People.* Bristol: The Policy Press.

Clarke, C. and Heyman, B. (1998) 'Risk management for people with dementia.' In B. Heyman (ed) *Risk, Health and Health Care.* London: Arnold.

Daker-White, G., Beattie, A., Means, R. and Gilliard, J. (2002) *Serving the Needs of Marginalised Groups in Dementia Care.* Bristol: University of West of England.

Department of Health (1998) *Modernising Social Services.* London: Department of Health.

Department of Health (2001) *National Service Framework for Older People.* London: Department of Health.

Elliott, A. (2002) 'Beck's sociology of risk: a critical assessment.' *Sociology 36,* 2, 293–315.

Giddens, A. (1999) *BBC Reith Lectures, The Runaway World.* London: BBC online.

Gilmour, H., Gibson, F. and Campbell, J. (2003) 'Living alone with dementia: a case study approach to understanding risk.' *Dementia 2,* 2, 245–264.

Herring, R. and Thom, B. (1997) 'The right to take risks: alcohol and older people.' *Social Policy and Administration 31,* 3, 233–246.

Kemshall, H. (2002) *Risk, Social Policy and Welfare.* Buckingham: Open University Press.

Law Commission (1997) *Who Decides? Decisions on Behalf of Mentally Incapacitated Adults.* London: The Law Commission.

Manthorpe, J. (2003) 'Risk and dementia: models for community mental health nursing practice.' In J. Keady, C.L. Clarke and T. Adams (eds) *Community Mental Health Nursing and Dementia Care: Practice Perspectives.* Buckingham: Open University Press/McGraw-Hill Education.

Marshall, M. (1984) 'Strategies for planning a better future for carers.' In Age Concern/Scotland *The Slow Death of the Intellect.* Edinburgh: Age Concern Scotland.

Martin, W. and Bartlett, H. (2003) 'Valuing people with dementia.' In T. Adams and J. Manthorpe (eds) *Dementia Care.* London: Arnold.

Misselbrook, D. and Armstrong, D. (2002) 'Thinking about risk. Can doctors and patients talk the same language?' *Family Practice 19,* 1–2.

Parker, G. (1993) *With This Body.* Buckingham: Open University Press.

Phillips, Lord (2000) *The BSE Inquiry, Volume 1, Findings and Conclusions.* London: The Stationery Office.

Simpson, R. and Simpson, A. (1999) *Through the Wilderness of Alzheimer's: A Guide in Two Voices.* Minneapolis, MN: Augsburg Fortress Publishers.

Snyder, L. (1999) *Speaking Our Minds: Personal Reflections from Individuals with Alzheimer's.* New York: W.H. Freeman and Co.

Social Services Inspectorate (1989) *Inspection of Community Social Services for Elderly People with Mental Disorder.* London: Department of Health.

Stalker, K. (2003) 'Managing risk and uncertainty in social work.' *Journal of Social Work 3,* 2, 211–234.

Strategy Unit (2002) *Risk: Improving Government's Capability to Handle Risk and Uncertainty.* London: Cabinet Office Strategy Unit.

Wilkinson, H. (ed) (2002) *The Perspectives of People with Dementia: Research Methods and Motivations.* London: Jessica Kingsley Publishers.

PART 4

*Representations
and Re-Presentations
of People with Dementia*

CHAPTER 10

Top-Dogs and Under-Dogs: Marginalising Problematic Voices[1]

Rik Cheston

This chapter is about how people with dementia change – more precisely it is about those emotional and social changes that occur in the time-limited psychotherapy groups that I have been running off and on for the last nine or ten years. For want of a better phrase I want to discuss how people with dementia 'come to terms with' their diagnosis.

Before I can move on and talk about how the people with dementia that I work with change, I need to talk about the process of change within psychotherapy. In more general terms this is also a model of the process of emotional change that we are all involved in as we struggle to adjust to changes and developments in our own lives.

The model of change that I have been using comes from psychotherapy process research – which as the name suggests is the form of research that looks at what happens in psychotherapy, regardless of the therapeutic orientation of the therapist involved, rather than at the outcome of that psychotherapy.

The model that I have been using to look at the change that occurs within our groups is called the Assimilation model developed by William Stiles and colleagues (e.g. Honos-Webb, Lani and Stiles 1999; Stiles *et al.* 1992, 1995, 1999). The central concern in the Assimilation model of psychotherapeutic change is the process by which painful or problematic experiences are gradually assimilated into existing schema. During the developmental process involved in ordinary learning, experiences are assimilated into existing beliefs or schemas, which in turn are altered to accommodate existing material. Problematic experiences are those which, were they to be assimilated in this way, would be psychologically painful. Instead these experiences are pushed away out of conscious awareness, although knowledge of their presence may leak back in the form of symptoms of psychological distress: for example, outbursts of anger, panic attacks or depression.

The Assimilation model proposes that the process by which problematic experiences are assimilated in successful psychotherapy involves clients moving through a series of stages or levels, as the painful material is approached, the nature of the problem clarified, insight gained and then mastery over the material achieved. As the problematic material is gradually assimilated into existing schema, so the client experiences a parallel sequence of emotional reactions. A client might move from being oblivious or feeling only vaguely disturbed, to experiencing the content first as painful and then as problematic but less distressing. In the later stages of this process, as the problem is understood and new solutions are tried out, so confidence grows and the client may gain some satisfaction or positive affect from the new way of living (Newman and Beail 2002).

The Assimilation model provides a way of understanding how clients within psychotherapy move from being unaware of the problematic material (or to put it another way 'in denial'), through a process of exploration and problem identification, to eventual understanding and insight that permits a wider problem-solving approach and final mastery of the problematic experience. This movement through a series of stages is operationalised through the Assimilation of Problematic Experiences Scale (or APES) shown in Table 10.1.

Research using assimilation analysis has focused on client, therapist and observer-defined insight events to trace these stages of assimilation. Recently the model has been applied to changes in awareness that occur during psychotherapy for individuals with intellectual disabilities (Newman and Beail 2002). In each case therapy has moved the individual along the scale without necessarily reaching stage seven, emphasising that the process of change is dependent on a multiplicity of individual factors. This highlights an important benefit of the Assimilation model: it is sensitive to change based on the individual's needs rather than the nature of the intervention or therapist; therefore, it is potentially applicable in a variety of settings.

Discursive interpretations

Assimilation analysis is a trans-theoretical model of the process of change that occurs within psychotherapy. As such it can be interpreted in terms of many

Table 10.1 Assimilation of Problematic Experiences Scale (APES)

APES level	Content	Affect
0. Warded off	Uninformed, unaware avoidance	Minimal affect, reflecting successful avoidance
1. Unwanted thoughts	Emergence of thoughts associated with discomfort	Unfocused strong emotions (e.g. anxiety, fear, sadness)
2. Vague awareness	Problematic experience is acknowledged and uncomfortable associated thoughts are described	Affect focused on acute psychological pain or panic
3. Problem statement or clarification	Clear problem statement	Negative but manageable affect
4. Understanding/ insight	Problem is formulated within a schema including clear connective links	Curiosity of affect, with mixed pleasant and unpleasant recognitions
5. Application/ working through	Working on current problem with reference to specific problem-solving efforts	Business-like positive/negative affect linked to outcomes
6. Problem solution	Success with a specific problem	Positive satisfaction linked to accomplishments
7. Mastery	Generalisation through habitual use of problem solution in new situations	Neutral (i.e. this is no longer something to get excited about)

formulations of therapy. Postmodern theories of the self describe a 'community of voices' rather than one, ever-present self; there are a series of 'selves' which are context-dependent, shifting and multiple (Hermans and Kempen 1992). In such a social constructionist perspective, problematic experiences develop because a dominant or 'top-dog' voice actively and successfully opposes the integration of an under-dog voice into the community of voices – instead the problematic voice is pushed away.

The top-dog voice can be understood as the voice of continuity, or the preservation of the status quo – it is a powerful voice because it is a voice of certainty, of the need to resist change. Often it is a voice which has the pretence of being unemotional, of emphasising the importance of control, of logic and of disallowing the vaguer expression of emotional unease.

The under-dog voice can be thought of as the voice of change – that something, somehow is wrong; that things are not as they should be, and that change is either necessary or unavoidable. It is the voice of uncertainty, of emotional hesitancy – perhaps it may be the voice of fear pointing towards a threat. At other times it is the voice of sadness and loss – that something is missing and needs to be grieved for. It can be the voice of embarrassment and of shame, or of self-reproach.

To give an example of this metaphor of voices: I have recently been mulling over whether to change jobs, which would involve moving from living near Bath to Norwich. In this process of change there are many voices, some arguing the need for change, others suggesting that life is just fine for both myself and my family just as we are. There is a debate, ever changing, yet always going over the same ground, as to whether change is needed or necessary.

Assimilation can be understood as a process in which a dialogue between the problematic voice, or under-dog, and the community of voices gradually arises, so that a shared meaning begins to form (Honos-Webb and Stiles 1998). In social constructionist terms, then, assimilation is represented as an alteration in the balance of voices – the problematic, under-dog voice strives for expression, but is at first warded off or successfully opposed by the dominant voice. This voice is then approached, allowed to be relevant, and finally accepted into the community of voices.

In order for this process to be allowed to happen – for the problematic experience to be assimilated – then the under-dog voice has to be heard. But this is a painful voice – not only may the person themselves not want to hear it, but others around that person too may not be able to hear it.

In the remainder of this chapter I want to look at the process of change that occurred for one man, Robert, in one ten-week group that I ran for people with dementia. The key event in allowing Robert to change, I will argue, was a session in which he challenged other members of the group, saying 'I don't think anyone here has got Alzheimer's disease'. In response to his challenge other group members replied, talking about their feelings of shame, loss and fear. This enabled his top-dog voice to listen to the under-dog voices.

The Dementia Voice Group Psychotherapy Project

This project involved establishing six psychotherapy groups across the south of England for people who had been diagnosed with Alzheimer's disease or another form of dementia. Each group lasted for ten weeks and was facilitated by the author in collaboration with either one or two co-facilitators who varied from group to group.

Participants

In all 42 people took part in the groups, all of whom were assessed as having either a mild or a moderate level of dementia. Most people lived at home with their husband or wife, although some lived on their own or in nursing care. All of the participants had a MMSE (Mini Mental State Examination) score of 18 or above, indicating that they had a mild or moderate level of cognitive impairment.

Therapeutic aims

The central aim of these groups was to bring people with dementia together to talk about 'what it's like when your memory doesn't work as well as it used to do'. Participants were encouraged to share their experiences with each other and to discuss the emotional impact of these experiences on them.

The need to listen and to bear witness

The counselling approach adopted by the facilitators within the groups was Resolution Therapy, a form of therapeutic intervention specifically developed for work with people with dementia (Stokes and Goudie 1990). Based on humanistic ideas of counselling, Resolution Therapy focuses on the importance of identifying the often hidden emotional message underlying the actions and language used by people with dementia and sensitively reflecting these back to them. This can be an effective way of helping people with dementia to make sense of what has been happening to them. A fuller description of the use of this style of working within a group setting with people with dementia can be found elsewhere (Cheston 1998; Cheston and Jones 2002; Cheston, Jones and Gilliard 2003a).

Changes in levels of depression and anxiety

Analysis of data collected independently of the facilitators of those 19 participants who completed the baseline, intervention and follow-up phases of the project provided significant evidence for a treatment effect lowering levels of depression and a strong trend towards a reduction in levels of anxiety. This change was maintained at follow-up and was independent of any effects of medication (Cheston, Jones and Gilliard 2003b). However, although it is important to be able to look at large-scale group trends, it is also vital to have some idea of how people change within sessions. In order to do this, we looked in detail at material gathered from one of the six groups, a process that is described in Watkins *et al.* (2002).

Analysis of the data

Audiotapes and data collected from the ten sessions of one of the six groups in this project were used for this analysis. The analysis presented here draws on methodology outlined by Stiles and his colleagues (e.g. Stiles 2000, 2001; Stiles *et al.* 1992, 1994, 1995, 1999; see also Newman and Beail 2002).

PHASE A: IDENTIFYING THEMES AND MAPPING INTERACTIONS

This involved working from the initial transcripts and tapes, so that each session was reviewed and re-reviewed until individual and group themes were identified. Written summaries were then made of the content of the group discussions, and the interactions between participants and facilitators. Changes in group-themes across the sessions were then mapped in relation to group processes.

PHASE B: DEFINING THE PROBLEMATIC EXPERIENCE

We decided to analyse material relating to a single participant who before the group began did not acknowledge having a diagnosis of Alzheimer's disease. The participant that we chose to examine was Robert, who attended all but one of the sessions. Robert was a 76-year-old retired solicitor who lived with his wife. He had received a diagnosis of dementia of the Alzheimer's type six months prior to the first session and, although he talked about his frustrations at his inability to remember, he was described as using denial as a means of coping.

The summaries and transcripts for each session were reviewed, highlighting Robert's descriptions of himself, his memory and, where relevant, his diagnosis. Five passages were identified in which Robert referred to his memory and to Alzheimer's disease. The two raters identified a number of common elements to these extracts which related to difficulties that Robert had in accepting the diagnosis of Alzheimer's disease. From this they formulated the following statement of the problematic experience: 'Robert coming to terms with the implications of his diagnosis of Alzheimer's disease.'

PHASE C: RATING THE LEVEL OF ASSIMILATION

Each of the five passages that related to the problematic experience were presented on audiotape and with detailed transcripts to an independent team of raters, none of whom had previously been involved in any aspect of the research, but who had received some training in the use of APES. The five passages were presented in a random order, and the researchers were asked to separately rate each extract within the passages using APES. When all the extracts had been presented and separately rated by the research group, the three analysts were then asked to listen to the extracts again and to discuss their ratings with each other so that they could reach a consensus rating for each extract. To enable fine gradations to be made between different extracts that were classified as being in the same category, ratings could be made from 0.1 to 0.9 in each category.

Week one

The first session began with a simple round of introductions, followed by the facilitators reminding participants about the purpose of the group. Robert defined his difficulty as a selective problem of short-term memory loss, which did not affect other areas of living, but was confined to a poor memory for finding his car, meeting people and so on.

> Robert: That's my big problem, in terms of method and getting on and doing, living and so on, I don't have any real problems, I don't find. But this problem of going places, doing things and meeting people and so on, I completely forget.

After a brief interruption, Robert then goes on to talk about a club that he belongs to, and in so doing makes the first reference in the group to Alzheimer's disease.

> Robert: Because everyone is in the same age bracket and half of them have got Alzheimer's or something near so we've all worked out ways of reminding each other in the conversation. You don't just

stand up and say something; you lead into it so other people know what they are doing.

Although Robert introduces the phrase 'Alzheimer's or something near' he does so in the context of distancing himself from it by using the phrase 'half of them'. Later on in the session he talks about finding strategies in the group to cope with the short-term memory loss, and to 'stimulate other parts of the brain to find passages through' to 'get a better memory system'. This sequence was rated as 0.1 ('warded off') because, although Robert does talk about having a memory problem and does not resist attempts to introduce it into the conversation, he positions Alzheimer's disease as something that affects other people and not him. Similarly, by searching for a solution, so it appears that he's actively avoiding greater awareness about his condition.

Week four

At the start of the session there was some discussion about the difficulties that people with Alzheimer's disease face. This discussion does not involve Robert, who listens before interrupting:

David: I think my brother has made it very clear to me that it's not going to be clever to, to try to drive your car when you've got Alzheimer's, because if you do have, have a prang or something like that.

Janet: You have what?

David: You have a prang.

Jenny: An accident.

David: And if that happens, someone's going to come along and say, 'Oh, you've got Alzheimer's, have you? Ah…'

Robert: You keep saying you have Alzheimer's, has that been formally diagnosed, because it's not the same thing as memory loss, you know.

Later in the session the group returns to discuss the difficulties that people with Alzheimer's face, and once again Robert interjects a question addressed to other participants.

David: What worries me is that there's some people who do get a bit mad and who say, 'I'm not going to go in the water if they've got people here who are Alzheimer's.'

Janet: Well they don't know what it means.

David: Of course they don't.

Janet: It's up to us as members of the Alzheimer's Society to have as much publicity as we can.

David: Absolutely.

Janet: And that will bring out a lot of people I think, a lot of people who have been ashamed of it. And for ashamed I mean there's all sorts of variants on that. And I think it would be a very good thing if there was, because a lot of people are frightened they've got it, or maybe they've been told and then they think it's shameful. And they, they feel isolated. So I think it's somehow, and I don't know what Alzheimer's Society policy is, but to make it like having a cold.

Facilitator: I'd like to just ask other people.

Janet: Sorry?

Facilitator: Well, I'd just like to put that to other people, Janet was saying that there's been a sort of shame about having Alzheimer's.

Janet: Oh yes, if you look throughout…

Keith: Yes, I do.

Janet: …at older people you love, like grandparents, they've had all sorts of things.

Keith: I wouldn't really want to, at the moment I wouldn't really want to let other people know.

Judith: No.

Robert: Now there's a premise here that I just don't agree with. The way you're talking, you sound as though you've accepted the fact that you've got Alzheimer's. Now I don't think anyone in this room has got Alzheimer's.

In response to this, four other members of the group who had previously been relatively quiet all acknowledged both that they too had been diagnosed as having Alzheimer's disease, and that they found this diagnosis unsettling and disturbing in some way. While some talked about it being embarrassing, and others about it being shameful, Judith spoke of her fears about the future:

Judith: I just wonder where it's all going to end, that's my fear…

Janet: When it's going to end?

Judith: *Where* it's going to end, where am I going to end up, just before the end, you know.

Janet: Oh, I see, you mean, I talk about death…

Judith: Yeah.

Janet: …to my family and I think the only thing that I'm frightened of is the unknown and that is death to me.

Judith: And after that. Oh, no I'm worried about what comes just before [laughs], it could be years before, couldn't it?

Janet: It could be tomorrow.

Robert: Is it the dying that?

Judith: I don't feel that at all, no, because we all go through that, no I'm not frightened about that, *no*. It's not really my religion to say it at all, but I don't know if there's anything else and I'm not going to worry about that right now, you know.

Facilitator: So what is the frightening, when you say about the future?

Judith: Being, being *useless*, you know.

Janet: Yes.

Judith: Not having all my faculties, I dread that, I dread that, it's as if I'm going to come to it one morning, perhaps, you know and think 'oh my godfathers, what's left?', I really worry about that…so I'm quite happy in a situation unless I choose to sort of sit there and think. And it's when I think about that, that the curtain comes down.

We have a range of different voices here: the voices of survivors (Janet, David) and the voice of a questioner, the top-dog voice of Robert. But there are also other voices enacted within the group: the voice of Keith and his concern that this is 'not something I'd wish to publicise' – of another in the group who said it was 'unfortunate that you've got it'.

Most clearly of all there is the voice of Judith – of her fears for the future of being 'completely useless', and of her need at that point to stop thinking, to allow the curtain to come down.

Week five

At the start of the session, Robert produces a piece of paper from his pocket on which he had written down thoughts from the previous week. He begins to talk about how he believes that the previous week's discussion had been based around a misconception:

> Robert: What I'm trying to say is that whatever problem a person has we all work the same way, we analyse that problem and we decide the relationship that it has with other events. And when we sum up all of those pieces together we come to a conclusion about what's the right way to go. Now that's the way that we solve problems. But to do that we very often have to rely on our experience. And our experience is either in deep memory or it's in short-term memory. Now the problem with Alzheimer's *as it affects me* is that I have no problems with retrieving the information in the long term.

This extract was rated by the consensus group as being 2.0 ('vague awareness') as, although Robert refers to himself as having Alzheimer's disease, he does not develop this statement. He is still negotiating with himself about whether this is a process of normal ageing and there is no direct acknowledgement of this problem as either being more widespread than a loss of short-term memory, or as part of a progressive illness. Shortly after this extract, Robert defines his problems further:

> Robert: All I'm trying to say is that there's no relationship, and I believe that in these meetings we've had a certain suggestion, perhaps subtle suggestion, has been implied that if the intelligence goes down, the short-term memory goes down *and* if the short-term memory goes down, the intelligence goes down...

Robert's affect during this extract becomes increasingly angry, and he speaks about himself being frustrated and angry. In part the anger seems to be directed against other members of the group whom he states have associated Alzheimer's disease with a loss of intelligence, in part with the group facilitators whom he says should have helped the group to find ways around his problems of short-term memory loss. This second extract from the session was rated as being 1.6 ('unwanted thoughts') – a stage that is characterised, in part, by a significant rise in affect and by a fear of losing control.

Week seven

Once again, Robert begins to talk at the start of the session, this time in a relaxed and humorous way:

> Robert: Can I tell you something that's happened to me in this last week. I've had a CT scan, which was quite an interesting thing in itself, but I got the results back yesterday and it said that my brain had shrunk very, very slightly in the cavity, which is fairly symptomatic of the onset of Alzheimer's. So I asked, 'Well if it's the *onset*, what happens when you're there' [group laughs], when you're there, and he said 'very little more'. I mean if you got to the point where you couldn't remember anything at all then the brain wouldn't have got any smaller but it's this shrinkage which brings about this symptom of short-term memory loss, which is quite intriguing. So I'm not particularly bothered by it, but it was interesting to go through it.

And later on he commented:

> Facilitator: I was just thinking, Robert, you said very calmly that you had the scan and they told you your brain had shrunk.
>
> Robert: It's still twice as big as everyone else's [group laughs] so it's quite all right. I was quite surprised about that, I didn't realise that the brain was an organ that could actually shrink. I don't think any other bones can shrink, but I don't think any other main part of the body can shrink.
>
> Judith: I think they do [laughs].

By contrast to the antagonism of the week five passage, Robert praised other members of the group, including Julie, whom he believed had 'got to grips with the problem more than anyone else'. At the same time there is a slightly manic element to Robert's response as if he still found it hard to take the impact of the diagnosis seriously. It was this affect and Robert's statements that 'I'm not particularly bothered by it' which influenced the consensus group to rate the extracts in this passage as 3.9 ('problem clarification') rather than as the following stage of 'problem understanding or insight'.

Week nine

The final sessions centred around issues relating to the ending of the group: for instance, how participants could support each other in the future.

Participants also took comfort in the group's ability to reduce feelings of being misunderstood and stigmatised. In the ninth session Robert reflected upon how he had changed over the course of the group:

Janet: You have to face it to start with.

Robert: Well I think that's inevitable, we wouldn't be here if we didn't do that. And so once we've accepted it, you need help from other people, you need help from yourselves, and we need help from groups like this. I find I've, I've got a great deal of moral uplift by coming here. Meeting you, listening to the way you do it. And I don't see the problem now, it frightened me, the problem of declining memory, until I came here, and now I'm not frightened.

Janet: You didn't accept it then before?

Robert: Well I did accept it but it frightened me. Because I thought, well, I'm going mad, I'm going crazy. What am I going to be like in another five years? But now I realise that everybody is getting this problem.

As this extract did not specifically mention the term 'Alzheimer's disease', it did not meet the criteria that we had set out for extracts to be rated by the research group. However, in reflecting on his experiences during the group and in describing a process of acceptance and a lowered level of anxiety Robert appears to be describing a process of change with many similarities to the APES model that we have used here.

Listening to the many voices of a person with dementia

Listening to the *voices* of people with dementia is a complex task. Enabling all the varied voices to be heard enables people to change – that, for me, is how psychotherapy occurs, so long as we do it often enough and sensitively enough by using the right word in the right place at the right time.

This means that we have to listen, facilitate or enable the right word, the right voice, to be heard – even when the right voice for that time is an uncomfortable voice, a distressing or pained voice.

Sometimes we can articulate this voice ourselves – in the context of group work it is more often the case that other members in the group articulate the under-dog voice. But to allow these voices to be articulated, so we have to listen to our own voices – of what we would like to think ourselves to be.

We risk presenting certain voices because they're easier to hear – we risk re-presenting people with dementia as survivors rather than as victims, because it helps us to hang on to hope.

How often have I heard people say that when it is the turn of my generation something to the effect that 'brought up on rebellion, on punk rock and human rights, then we won't crack – we will demand our entitlements'. That may be so, but there is another voice inside me that says that maybe I would not be brave enough to do that, maybe there won't be anyone else to hear me. I do not know if I will be braver, more courageous than my grandfather: he had Alzheimer's disease – he fought throughout the First World War as a sergeant in the Gloucestershire Regiment. He fought on the Somme, and in the Balkans. For saving the life of his injured captain under enemy fire he was awarded the Military Medal. Yet as an old man I recall he went quietly along, didn't assert his knowledge of what was happening to him. Should I dare to think that should I develop Alzheimer's disease, then I will be braver than him in facing my future? Will any of my generation be more assertive than those who have gone before us when, and if, it is our time?

But it is not just the possible future that makes these voices problematic, that makes it hard to hear, it is also the present.

In some ways it is easier to hear the voice of Janet than of Judith in the fourth week. Janet was often able to speak openly about her illness. Her commanding voice offers hope for the future – part of me would like to feel that if, God forbid, one day it may be my turn to have Alzheimer's, then I too may be as assertive, strong and adamant as Janet was that my illness should be no more an embarrassment to me than having a cold.

But there is another voice within me, that, like Judith, I too would be frightened and fearful of becoming completely useless. At another point in the sessions Judith talked about her shame of avoiding a woman in her block of flats who crept slowly and pitifully along the hallway, calling for help. Judith was ashamed of herself, saying that she used to be a teacher and that she used to think of herself as being the first to offer help to others. Now she told the group that she hides away and avoided coming out.

The reason that I am, inside, more sure that I would be more like Judith than like Janet is because I know that even now I am ashamed of myself at times. There are times when I choose not to hear patients calling out in the ward where I work, where I avoid eye contact because I don't want to be called on, because I have work to do, because it's someone else's job, not mine, because I'm too tired, because sometimes I'm afraid that I can't do it any more.

Knowing that Judith's voice already reverberates uncomfortably inside me makes it harder for me to hear what she has to say. In the group I didn't really know what to say for her. It is only now, on reflection, that I am really beginning to understand this.

However, if we only anticipate a single voice, or if we can only allow some voices and not others (the voice of survivors for instance, because they are more comfortable for us to hear), then we risk disallowing other voices – the voices of shame and embarrassment, or the voice of a frightened victim.

If we cannot allow these voices to be heard, then we cannot help people to change. Robert could only change, I would argue, because he heard others speak the voices that he himself could not.

Alzheimer's disease and the other dementias are uniquely evil, uniquely challenging – because they may be lying in wait for us in our lives. They challenge us to accept our own mortality, our own inadequacies. Unless we hear our own voices, about how we deal with our own, personal challenges, then we cannot hear the voices of those we work with.

In the context of this publication, I would argue that we risk marginalising some voices because they're too painful for us to hear – we hear them already in our work, in our lives, as we think (or try not to think, like Judith) about how we shall be when it is our turn, if it is to be our turn.

Note

1   The research on which this chapter is based was supported by a grant from the Mental Health Foundation and from Avon and Wiltshire Mental Health Partnership.

References

Cheston, R. (1998) 'Psychotherapeutic work with people with dementia: a review of the literature.' *British Journal of Medical Psychology 71*, 3, 211–231.

Cheston, R. and Jones, K. (2002) 'A place to work it all out together.' In S. Benson (ed) *Dementia Topics for the Millennium and Beyond.* London: Hawker Publications.

Cheston, R., Jones, K. and Gilliard, J. (2003a) 'Forgetting and remembering: group psychotherapy with people with dementia.' In T. Adams and J. Manthorpe (eds) *Dementia Care.* London: Edward Arnold.

Cheston, R., Jones, K. and Gilliard, J. (2003b) 'Group psychotherapy and people with dementia.' *Aging and Mental Health 7*, 6, 452–461.

Hermans, H. and Kempen, H. (1992) 'The dialogical self: beyond individualism and rationalism.' *American Psychologist 47*, 23–33.

Honos-Webb, L. and Stiles, W. (1998) Reformulation of assimilation analysis in terms of voices.' *Psychotherapy 35*, 1, 23–33.

Honos-Webb, L., Lani, J. and Stiles, W. (1999) 'Discovering markers of assimilation stages: the fear of losing control marker.' *Journal of Clinical Psychology 55*, 12, 1441–1452.

Newman, D. and Beail, N. (2002) 'Monitoring change in psychotherapy with people with intellectual disabilities: the application of the Assimilation of Problematic Experiences Scale.' *Journal of Applied Research in Intellectual Disabilities 15*, 48–60.

Stiles, W. (2000) *Assimilation Analysis*. Workshop, SPR-UK, Ravenscar, North Yorkshire, UK.

Stiles, W. (2001) 'The Assimilation Model.' Paper presented at *Towards Understanding Psychotherapeutic Processes*. Conference, Ulm, 2001.

Stiles, W., Honos-Webb, L. and Lani, J. (1999) 'Some functions of narrative in the assimilation of problematic experiences.' *Journal of Clinical Psychology 55*, 10, 1213–1226.

Stiles, W., Meshot, C., Anderson, T. and Sloan, W. (1992) 'Assimilation of problematic experiences: the case of John Jones.' *Psychotherapy Research 2*, 2, 81–101.

Stiles, W., Shapiro, D. and Harper, H. (1994) 'Finding the way from process to outcome.' In R. Russell (ed) *Reassessing Psychotherapy Research*. London: The Guilford Press.

Stiles, W., Shapiro, D., Harper, H. and Morrison, L. (1995) 'Therapist contributions to psychotherapeutic assimilation: an alternative to the drug metaphor.' *British Journal of Medical Psychology 68*, 1–13.

Stokes, G. and Goudie, F. (1990) 'Counselling confused elderly people.' In G. Stokes and F. Goudie (eds) *Working with People with Dementia*. Bicester, Oxon: Winslow.

Watkins, B., Cheston, R., Jones, K. and Gilliard, J. (2002) 'Emotional change within a psychotherapeutic group for people with dementia.' *PSIGE Annual Conference*, 10–12 July, King Alfred's College, Winchester.

CHAPTER 11

Images, Constructs, Theory and Method: Including the Narrative of Dementia

Gillian McColgan

Introduction

Despite a definitive research focus on finding the social meaning of dementia developed over the last decade, lack of understanding and negative popular representations of dementia persist. These impact directly upon people who have dementia and their families. When people are labelled as having dementia, and additionally live in a nursing home, negative attributions and a disabling environment result. These issues provide the context for research findings from an ethnographic study conducted in a private nursing home for people with dementia.

My research fieldwork took place in Lavender Wing of Deer View Grange Nursing Home[1] during nine months in 1999. Lavender Wing housed 12 residents in individual bedrooms with en-suite bathrooms and shared public rooms and corridors. Nine of these residents became research informants in this study. Fieldwork consisted of participant observation and taped interviews with residents, which took place almost exclusively in the public rooms of the Grange.

In this chapter I will explore popular representations, images, characterisations and attitudes to older people and people with dementia. Part of this will involve considering the impact of labelling someone as having dementia. Labelling of people in the Grange occurred merely by being a resident because the Grange was designated a dementia-specific nursing home. The particular culture of nursing homes will be established to show that, like the derogatory connotations of labelling, the environment can also disable those within.

Having set the context in which this study was undertaken I wish to take the lead from research participants in re-presenting dementia, that is by following their examples of reconstructing narratives to take account both of having dementia and of living in a nursing home. My re-presentation of dementia is based on an appropriate theoretical perspective and methodology, which can help to include, rather than exclude, people with dementia. It is premised on putting the person first.

Representations of ageing and dementia

As Hepworth (2000) and Manthorpe (1996, 2000) have demonstrated, fiction can give clear indications of characterisations of older people and people with dementia which may 'guide' the reader 'towards a deeper understanding' (Hepworth 2000, p.16). In addition to fictional accounts such as those by Forster (1990) and Ignatieff (1994) there are accounts written by people in the early stages of having dementia (for example Davis 1984; McGowin 1993; Rose 1996) and those who have had someone close to them with dementia (Appignanesi 1999; Grant 1998). Oddly, these personal accounts, like the fictional ones, also characterise people with dementia and use stereotypical images. Thus fictionally 'Grandma' is seen as vulnerable and unable to cope (Forster 1990); a mother is reduced by her neurologist to a 'case study' and subject to loss and decline (Ignatieff 1994); and titles of personal accounts suggest journeys into dementia, being engulfed and lost, and longing to go home (Davis 1984; McGowin 1993; Rose 1996). These images only serve to illustrate how pervasive such representations are.

Popular images of dementia are also strongly influenced by and represented in the media and, as Gubrium (1986) pointed out, there have also been celebrity tragedies linked to Alzheimer's disease. He described how the story of Rita Hayworth's Alzheimer's became public knowledge through her daughter's campaigning which was aimed at promoting more research into the condition. Ironically, part of this campaigning targeted the US President at the time, Ronald Reagan, whose own subsequent Alzheimer's disease also became public knowledge. Other public figures have since spoken out about dementia and their own experiences. In 2003, Rikki Fulton, a popular Scottish comedian, was the focus of a documentary shown on BBC Scotland when Kirsty Wark interviewed him with his wife about living with Rikki's dementia

(Wark Clements 2003). Iris Murdoch's dementia was also documented in her husband's works (Bayley 1998, 1999). In a diary entry just over a year before she died he wrote:

> Every day we are physically closer; and Iris's little 'mouse cry'…seems less and less forlorn, more simple, more natural. She is not sailing into the dark: the voyage is over, and under the dark escort of Alzheimer's she has arrived somewhere. So have I. (Bayley 1998, p.183)

His books are about their evolving relationship which he saw as growing closer physically as Iris' mental capacity declined. The metaphorical journey featured is one often talked of in personal accounts of dementia, and the escort is 'dark'. This 'dark' journey suggests a trajectory of decline reflecting expectations of a model of disease.

Equally interesting to these very personal views of the experience of dementia are those popular characterisations demonstrated in the reports and obituaries following Iris Murdoch's death. An analysis of these showed dementia as the tragedy of the loss of mental capacity highlighted for someone known for her intellect. Descriptions were of descent, a dreadful trance-like state, of a clouded old age and of Iris being struck down, stricken and subjected to the dreaded knock of Professor Alzheimer. 'Some of the accounts portray the dementia in essentialist terms, suggesting that Iris was demented rather than that she had dementia' (McColgan, Valentine and Downs 2000, p.107).

The distinction between being demented or living with dementia is important for the way the person is perceived. Eyewitness accounts further highlight the pervasive image of the person being lost to the disease. Such characterisations have undoubtedly been fuelled by ageist assumptions, the medicalisation of dementia and also by the labelling of people with dementia.

Sociological literature on ageism is well established. Age, and particularly old age, is subject to characterisations and stereotyping 'constructed from a complex blend of discourse and sensory images' (Featherstone and Wernick 1995, p.5). When one group applies these stereotypical images to another it amounts to prejudice; when this is related to chronological age, it is ageism (Bytheway 1997, p.3). While ageism is not exclusive to old age, this is the main way in which the term is used.

Ageist assumptions about older people relate to moral panic and 'the dependency ratio', which is based upon economic activity and defined in terms of working ages. Thus people are defined as dependent when they are under 16 and over 64 years old (Bytheway 1997, p.52). However, children are seen as potential assets while older people are not. Blaikie (1999) points out that ageism arises both in social structures, as seen in policy, and in individual attitudes. These are legitimised by 'ideological supports' through 'biological reductionism', 'psychological explanations' and 'social justification', which deny rights, create dependency and suggest that older people 'want to disengage from society' (Blaikie 1999, p.17).

All of these are the ways in which others perceive older people, and since a sense of self is often defined by reflections from others, or relationally to them, then negative stereotypes can impact on self-image. However, inner consciousness and outer bodily appearance often conflict in old age. When we catch a glimpse of ourselves in a mirror we are often surprised by the image we see, that we do not outwardly appear as we feel inside. This has been described as the 'mask of ageing' (Featherstone and Hepworth 1988, 1990; Hepworth 1991), a description of the disparity between the 'inner' self and 'outer' projection. Ageist assumptions are constructed on the basis of our physical appearance: '…it is the ageing mask which is pathological or deviant and the inner essential self which remains – even beneath or "inside" Alzheimer's disease – as normal' (Featherstone and Hepworth 1988, p.379).

Negative stereotyping of old age is related to culturally valued images of youth which are specific both temporally and culturally (Featherstone and Hepworth 1990, p.274). Their specificity identifies them as socially constructed.

Dementia has also been shown to be socially constructed. Until the mid-1980s academic literature relating to dementia was dominated by the medical model which established dementia as a disease category set on a trajectory of linear decline. Initial questioning of the way the medical model pathologises dementia was made by Gubrium (1986). He debated whether Alzheimer's disease may be classified as a 'normal' part of ageing, and suggested that depending upon how neurological and behavioural evidence was presented it could support either a theory of ageing or of disease. This appears to be the first indication that dementia may be considered pathological as the result of labelling and also that dementia may be socially constructed.

A further indication of Alzheimer's disease being socially constructed came in Lyman's critique of the biomedicalisation of dementia (1989). She points out that Alzheimer's disease only 'emerged as an illness category and policy issue in the 1980s, more than 70 years after Alois Alzheimer documented the first case' (Lyman 1989, p.597). This was due to 'senility' being regarded as a normal part of ageing until this time.

The social construction of dementia serves the purpose of helping people make sense of the chaos of living with dementia (Gubrium 1986; Lyman 1989). It counters the 'longstanding ageist assumption that senility is an inevitable condition of old age' (Lyman 1989, p.599). Dementia is difficult to objectify or explain factually, which is why it is often introduced in alarming terms (Gubrium 1986, p.33). This alarm amounts to moral panic, a situation for which those subjected to negative characterisations are blamed.

I wish to return to the concept of the 'mask of age' (Hepworth 1991); that people as they age still feel the same as when they were younger and are shocked to see a mirror image of an older person. If we are to follow Gubrium's (1986) argument that dementia is a normal part of ageing, then dementia would be the ultimate and final mask of ageing. Dementia is pathologised, perhaps because it presents all the worst scenarios of ageing and correspondingly becomes the most exaggerated and easy target for ageism. This ageism can be the result of labelling someone with dementia.

Labelling serves different purposes for different parties. Carers may be seeking an explanation of unusual behaviour while people labelled as mentally ill may perceive collusion in the diagnosis procedure between family and health professionals (Goffman 1991). Diagnosis and labelling often offer an explanation of unusual behaviour for informal carers and family members.

The benefits of the label of 'dementia' are not so clear for people thus labelled as they are for their families. There is also a danger that, once labelled, all behaviour will be attributed to dementia. As Cheston and Bender point out 'a diagnosis identifies an individual as a member of a specific group of patients' (2000, p.50). They also say that 'the process whereby a diagnosis is reached is inevitably a subjective one carried out by fallible human beings' (p.50).

It has been shown that stereotyping of dementia and old age stigmatises older people with dementia, and that the views of old age differ from the subjective views of individuals. There is a disabling effect for each stigmatisation that compounds when someone is both old and has dementia. Once labelled, this may determine the 'career' (Goffman 1991) of the person. Labelling also has an effect in the attribution of all actions to the label; in this case to dementia. This impacts on self-image, and causes tensions between the inner and outer person. These tensions may become more pronounced with a move into residential care in which life becomes more public than private. In this sense the environment also has a disabling effect on the person who has dementia and finds themselves in unfamiliar surroundings. A discussion on the particular culture of nursing homes might help to clarify this.

Ethnographic studies of nursing homes which have appeared in the last 30 years suggest that there is a specific culture associated with nursing homes (for example Gubrium 1997; Lee-Treweek 1998; Savishinsky 1991), reflected upon in a collection of articles in *The Culture of Long Term Care* (Henderson and Vesperi 1995). The growth in this area of research corresponds with that of the field of gerontology, sparked by demographic changes and an ageing population (Coleman and Bond 1992). Combined, they can produce a negative image of ageing, giving rise to ageist assumptions of decline and dependency. I wish to argue that if older people and people with dementia living in nursing homes are considered to be a burden, a perspective that can arise from wider moral panic, the nursing home environment can often reinforce this image and reflect it back to society.

Through discourse, institutions such as nursing homes are able to reflect and reinforce dominant values in a collective way. A theoretical scheme develops which, when viewed in the context of this discourse, makes categorisation of even ambiguous elements appear natural and part of everyday life. Douglas (1986) suggests that through this process institutions virtually 'think', a constantly evolving procedure which accounts for the present and also (re)constructs the past to make it relevant to the present (Douglas 1986, p.69).

Studies of nursing homes reflect the culture and the continuing dominance of the medical model. As Savishinsky comments on the contradictory role of the nursing home, 'the home that could not be a home, and the medical facility that rarely restored people to health – derived from the fact that the institution was neither a proper home nor a hospital' (Savishinsky 1991, p.248). This contradiction is particularly important for people with dementia, where there is little prospect of treatment or cure.

In Deer View Grange bowel movements, appetites and moods were charted for each resident. Routines and regimens were dominant. Other studies also reflect nursing homes as a 'Cult of Time and Task' (Henderson 1995) with an emphasis on 'bed and body work' (Gubrium 1997, pp.123–57). Residents have frequently been infantilised (Hockey and James 1993; Lyman 1993) and treated as if they were children. This was also in evidence when staff were preparing for a Halloween party in Lavender Wing and one care assistant commented to me that it was like doing a party for the children. The culture, in addition to infantilisation, discouraged residents from being independent as there was little time for individuality; instead residents were efficiently presented in the lounge in a manner that Sabat (1994) described as encouraging excess disability – a form of over-dependence.

The nursing home culture of routine in the Grange was also one of surveillance as described in Goffman's (1991) 'Total Institutions' and in Foucault's (1991) 'Panopticons'. Both are characterised similarly as means to exert group control using minimal staffing. Such a system allows little opportunity for resident autonomy. Individuality also becomes subservient to the convenience of the group of people in the nursing home. Even when interests conflict, individuals may be expected to remain under the control of the limited staff members. This is highlighted by Goffman's description: '…under conditions where one person's infraction is likely to stand out in relief against the visible constantly examined compliance of the others' (Goffman 1991, p.18). Organising 'blocks' of people in this way thus allows easy detection of 'infractions'. As Foucault (1991) also pointed out, this ensures surveillance without the need for skilled workers.

The result of this nursing home culture for residents is one of complying to rules 'for their own good'. As Berger (1991) comments: 'Identity comes with conduct and conduct occurs in response to specific social situations' (p.119). Thus, in this way, the identity of residents is shaped by the specific social situation that arises from this nursing home culture. This culture can disable in the same way as disability studies have shown occurs for impaired people (Corker and French 1999).

In Lavender Wing of the Grange there was strong evidence of group control in the interests of maintaining minimal staffing levels. This inevitably meant that it was not easy to accommodate a wish for privacy or be away from the group as my fieldnotes recorded:

> Rebecca Jackson wandered the corridor for a good bit of my visit and I heard later from a care assistant that she had tried to lock herself in her room. 'She then just sat in her room and wouldn't come out.' Staff nurse said she wasn't upset at all, but the care assistant and staff nurse obviously thought this was odd behaviour.

Rebecca was carving out some privacy by crossing the 'boundaries between public and private places' (Gubrium 1997, p.3). By choosing to be in her designated private room, she was not easily controlled as part of the group. Within this surveillance culture, her behaviour was considered strange. Similarly another resident, Betty MacRobert, made frequent requests to be taken to her room to sleep. When I witnessed these requests it was usually during the afternoon. Betty had mobility difficulties and could not go to her room unaided. Each time I heard Betty ask to be taken to her room to sleep she was refused without reason. I believe that the refusals were given in the interests of maintaining group control through surveillance.

My research findings in Deer View Grange support other literature on specific nursing home cultures. In order for this culture to operate, residents are subjected to group control and stripped of individuality. Part of this process is in the application of characterisations, stereotypes and labelling of dementia, where the person appears totally consumed by the disease. However, even within the Grange there was evidence that this was not the reality. By a re-presentation of the evidence this should become apparent.

Reconstructing the self through narrative

Research informants in the Grange frequently told stories of their lives. In the telling, these stories were rehearsed, reinforced and reinterpreted through the narration of the story of self and others. When people have a lifetime of experiences behind them this is commonly done through the telling of life stories (Harré 1998; Holstein and Gubrium 2000). Even when the memories of recent events might falter with dementia, these residents were often able to recount details of events long past. Through their telling, they remained a part of the present and an important element of self-identity. With each retelling they reinforced and reconstructed this identity in the context of people's current circumstances. These accounts tell who the person is today by consistent construction of the past (Strauss 1997).

For research participants, narrating their life story gave an opportunity to present a particular history of their past. An argument made for disengagement in later life, a deliberate withdrawal from social life, suggests that some roles have been lost by the discontinuation of work (Cumming and Henry 1961). Narrative presents an opportunity to replace these lost roles and carve out an identity of who a person is now by saying who they had been, what they had experienced and what they had done during their lives.

Residents participating in this study had undergone many changes throughout their lives. Most recently, and common to all residents, these changes had related to ageing, the onset of dementia and the move to residential care. With each change an adjustment period will have taken place when redefinition of the self will have occurred. In much the same way as marriage redefines personal biographies in the context of the changed circumstance of the marriage (Berger and Kellner 1972), the self is (re)constructed in the context of ageing, dementia and changed living circumstances; that is, the past is reconstructed retrospectively to take account of current circumstances.

Accounts are transformed to explain these changes and passages of status (Strauss 1997).

In Isobel MacDonald's transformed accounts, people around her were defined as 'Italian' or 'Scots'. Isobel would narrate tales of her life in the forces, a time when she was apparently surrounded by many people, some of whom she knew well and others whom she did not. She recounted that she always got on with the Italians, but did not always understand them, pointing out someone in the room who was 'Italian'. Then she would continue to point out the 'Scots lassies', the ones she 'shared with', got on well with, and understood. One of the residents would spend long periods of the day groaning and calling for her 'daddy'. This often impacted on the mood of Lavender Wing and tended to promote confusion and chaos. On one such occasion, I was interviewing Isobel, who originated from Glasgow, and she asked me, 'Where is she from, Edinburgh? I cannae understand her.' The rivalry that exists between Glasgow and Edinburgh and the distinct identity for people from these places, something that Isobel would have been aware of her life, provided an explanation for her incomprehension of this resident.[2]

Drawing on her experiences from the past to make sense of the present shows how Isobel defined the situation. Place was part of Isobel's value system, narrated in life stories and accounted for in transformations. At no time was this more apparent than in a statement she made in which she said, 'I don't really want to be classed as just a person as this...I would rather be classed a different place.' Besides being about place, this statement was about control and choice and about Isobel trying to regain these in a disabling environment.

Another person who narrated stories of his past was Jimmy McLean. Often with bravado, tales were told of his drunken father who was a boxer, of work, of hardship and of camaraderie. Jimmy defined himself by what he had done: 'I've been all over the place. I've been all over the country, working, round the houses and that, digging, mining...never on the dole' [interview with Jimmy McLean].

This 'never on the dole' was said with pride, a clear defining feature of self-identity. Jimmy often puzzled over things that did not make sense to him and for which he sought explanation. I found that themes would recur in conversation over many days until an account was formulated. For instance, he puzzled over the chain of events that had led to him moving into the Grange. Gradually over several days he pieced together illnesses and accidents occurring when he lived alone culminating in a serious accident which caused him to be hospitalised for several months. After these events had been told to me, a new account emerged in which Jimmy chose to move into the Grange because he was 'fed up' with his own company. This became the narrative repeated to me on many other subsequent occasions.

Narratives of self reflect and reveal values held by the narrator. Alice Taylor was very concerned with her appearance, often checking a mirror during the day to see how she looked, and this was also manifested in her narrations of the past. She talked of her hair being long and put into ringlets, and confirmed the importance of having nice-looking hair by telling me of her regular visits to the hairdressers now. Within her accounts she very clearly spoke with voice, distinctly expressing how *she* imagined others perceived *her*: 'Always wee Alice, to everyone I was Alice. Everyone would come in the Plough, looking for wee Alice, where is she? I want to give her a hug' [interview with Alice Taylor].

Alice re-presented her popularity in her narrative. She also liked to reiterate that she was popular in the Grange and that she knew everyone. She told me that the lady sitting opposite her had worked in the 'Shell Factory' with her during the war and that they were really good friends reunited in the Grange. Whenever someone walked past, she told a story of her friendship with them, yet she rarely sat with other residents and had conversations mainly with staff, visitors and myself.

Research participants in this study narrated their lives and parts of their lives in interviews. Change in circumstances often initiated a retrospective reconstruction in relation to a new situation, such as occurs with married couples. Within marriage, personal histories are redefined in order to relate them to the partnership (Berger and Kellner 1972). The narration of self by residents of the Grange in the context of having dementia and of living in a nursing home meant that the self was re-constructed to take account of these changes. Often involving retrospective re-construction of the past, this was a complex process which helped to make sense of the present.

Re-presenting dementia

We could take the lead from people with dementia by re-presenting dementia today in a similar vein of re-constructing the past to take account of the present. Awareness of dementia is increasing and the current inclination of celebrities to make their experiences of dementia public is a part of this. These public declarations and accounts have raised awareness and understanding of dementias. By knowing that people we know and public figures that we often feel we know are not immune to dementias we get a sense of them being classless pollutants. Through this thinking it becomes conceivable that any of us might experience dementias, and like environmental risks beyond our individual control, dementia then becomes another risk that 'cares not a jot about the polluter pays principle' (Beck 1992, p.39). This context might provide enough impetus for us all to wish for consideration of the personhood of people with dementia.

A central concern of Kitwood's (1997) was personhood, in his aim to change the culture of care for people with dementia. Much of his work was concerned with trying to place a different value emphasis on dementia care and research, by changing the paradigm from one dominated by an 'organic mental disorder' to a 'new culture'. The concept of 'personhood' with which he wished us to regard people who have dementia 'is a standing or status that is bestowed upon one human being, by others, in the context of relationship and social being. It implies recognition, respect and trust' (Kitwood 1997, p.8). He pointed out that people with dementia have the same needs and rights as everyone else, and that we have a moral obligation to treat them with dignity and respect. Post echoed a similar opinion: 'Too great a value emphasis on rationality and memory…wrongly excludes people with dementia from the sphere of human dignity and respect' (Post 1995, p.2).

In order to theorise dementias and to acknowledge that those who have them should be treated with respect, dignity and trust, an appropriate theoretical perspective would be one which places the person before dementia. Such theory guided my fieldwork methods and interpretation of data and was based upon what it is like to experience everyday life in the social world.

Theories of everyday life have been used to consider how any people make sense of their social world and this is why I considered them appropriate for this study. This meant that it was the people living in Deer View Grange who were studied and the fact that my research participants also had dementia became almost incidental and secondary.

Through theories of everyday life interactions, emotions and categorisation skills were explored and, contrary to literature focusing on a medical model, were seen to be present. Research participants were also social participants engaging in interactions and social exchanges. They picked up on social cues (Strauss 1997, pp.48–9), co-operated with others to aid the flow of conversation (Goffman 1963, p.24) and engaged in turn-taking in conversation (Sacks, Schegloff and Jefferson 1974; Schegloff and Sacks 1973). They also engaged in farewells and leave-taking when I was to depart after a period of ethnographic study. I will give an example of this in greetings upon my arrival.

Throughout the fieldwork, I tried as much as possible to allow residents to approach me and to initiate interactions, with myself taking a more passive role in the relationships. Physical limitations of residents sometimes meant that I needed to take more initiative in the interactions. However, an ideal opportunity presented one morning when I arrived in Lavender Wing while residents were in the dining room eating breakfast. I sat and waited in the lounge silently and eventually residents started to make their way in, some independently and others with assistance from care staff. Although I played a totally passive role, not attempting to catch the eye of any resident, every one of the nine participants in the study went through the process of catching my eye and either speaking, nodding or smiling by way of greeting me. Alice Taylor and Jimmy McLean, with whom I would often sit and talk in the mornings, were even apologetic that they had not seen me straight away. This is consistent with Goffman's notion of social recognition:

> ...there is 'social recognition', namely, the process of openly welcoming or at least accepting the initiation of an engagement, as when a greeting or smile is returned...in order to carry out certain forms of social recognition it will be necessary for the participants to recognise each other cognitively, or affect having done so, or apologise for not doing so. (Goffman 1963, p.113)

This is exactly what I found residents did when I waited for their initiation of a welcome. It was a skill retained by all research participants, whether or not they had lost some language through dementia.

Careful selection of methods was one way in which these voices could be heard in the research process. Ethnography allowed time, depth of information and familiarity to be gathered. Reduction of the activity and initiation by the researcher allowed more active participation by research informants. My apparent passivity in the process gave time for initiation of interactions by residents, an opportunity each one of them took regardless of any communication difficulties, by welcoming me on arrival.

Conclusion

In this chapter I have discussed images, attitudes, stereotypes and characterisations of older people and of people with dementia through examination of fiction, personal accounts, of media representations and in nursing homes. Nursing homes stigmatise and prejudice those labelled by others. To discuss whether nursing homes are the appropriate place for people with dementias has been beyond the scope of this chapter – however, I have been able to illustrate how this environment reflects and reinforces negative attitudes.

Following Kitwood's lead and the lead of research participants (who were people with dementia) I have tried to show alternative ways in which older people and people with dementia could be viewed. Just as people with dementia reconstructed their pasts through narrative, I have attempted to reconstruct some of what it is to be a person with dementia. This has been done by an appropriate methodological and theoretical perspective, one which could be used to view *any* people, and thus place the persons before dementia. The result is not to deny or trivialise dementias, but to place them secondary to the person. By this emphasis, every interaction and action was not attributed to dementia but was part of the individuality of the person.

Re-presenting the narrative of dementia, as I have attempted to do in this chapter, is one way in which I see an inclusive future for people with dementias. A fundamental shift away from representations, characterisations, images, attitudes and stereotypes which show people as demented and towards people who also have dementia would greatly help with this change.

Notes

1   Pseudonyms are used for the setting and research participants to maintain anonymity.

2   On several occasions since this research was conducted when I have interviewed older people from Glasgow they have asked me if I am from Edinburgh when they have not fully understood what I have said.

References

Appignanesi, L. (1999) *Losing the Dead: A Family Memoir*. London: Chatto and Windus.

Bayley, J. (1998) *Iris: A Memoir of Iris Murdoch*. London: Duckworth.

Bayley, J. (1999) *Iris and the Friends: A Year of Memories*. London: Duckworth.

Beck, U. (1992) *Risk Society*. London: Sage.

Berger, P.L. (1991) *Invitation to Sociology: A Humanistic Perspective*. Harmondsworth: Penguin.

Berger, P.L. and Kellner, H. (1972) 'Marriage and the construction of reality: an exercise in the microsociology of knowledge.' In B.R. Cosin, I.R. Dale, G.M. Esland, D. Mackinnon and D.F. Swift (eds) *School and Society: A Sociological Reader*, 2nd edition. London and Henley: Routledge and Kegan Paul.

Blaikie, A. (1999) *Ageing and Popular Culture*. Cambridge: Cambridge University Press.

Bytheway, B. (1997) *Ageism*. Buckingham: Open University Press.

Cheston, R. and Bender, M. (2000) *Understanding Dementia: The Man with the Worried Eyes.* London: Jessica Kingsley Publishers.

Coleman, P. and Bond, J. (1992) 'Ageing in the twentieth century.' In J. Bond and P. Coleman (eds) *Ageing in Society: An Introduction to Social Gerontology.* London: Sage.

Corker, M. and French, S. (1999) 'Reclaiming discourse in disability studies.' In M. Corker and S. French (eds) *Disability Discourse.* Buckingham: Open University Press.

Cumming, E. and Henry, W. (1961) *Growing Old: The Process of Disengagement.* New York: Basic Books.

Davis, R. (1984) *My Journey into Alzheimer's Disease.* Illinois: Tyndale.

Douglas, M. (1986) *How Institutions Think.* Syracuse: Syracuse University Press.

Featherstone, M. and Hepworth, M. (1988) 'The mask of ageing and the postmodern life course.' In M. Featherstone, M. Hepworth and B.S. Turner (eds) (1995) *The Body: Social Process and Cultural Theory.* London: Sage.

Featherstone, M. and Hepworth, M. (1990) 'Images of ageing.' In J. Bond and P. Coleman (eds) (1992) *Ageing in Society: An Introduction to Social Gerontology.* London: Sage.

Featherstone, M. and Wernick, A. (1995) *Images of Aging: Cultural Representations of Later Life.* London: Routledge.

Forster, M. (1990) *Have the Men Had Enough?* Harmondsworth: Penguin.

Foucault, M. (1991) *Discipline and Punish: The Birth of the Prison.* Harmondsworth: Penguin.

Goffman, E. (1963) *Behaviour in Public Places: Notes on the Social Organization of Gatherings.* London: Free Press.

Goffman, E. (1991) *Asylums: Essays on the Social Situation of Mental Patients and Other Inmates.* Harmondsworth: Penguin.

Grant, L. (1998) *Remind Me Who I Am, Again.* London: Granta Books.

Gubrium, J. (1986) *Oldtimers and Alzheimer's: The Descriptive Organisation of Senility.* London: JAI Press.

Gubrium, J. (1997) *Living and Dying at Murray Manor.* New York: St Martin's Press.

Harré, R. (1998) *The Singular Self: An Introduction to the Psychology of Personhood.* London: Sage.

Henderson, J.N. (1995) 'The culture of care in a nursing home: effects of a medicalised model of long term care.' In J.N. Henderson and M.D. Vesperi (eds) *The Culture of Long Term Care: Nursing Home Ethnography.* London: Bergin and Garvey.

Henderson, J.N. and Vesperi, M.D. (eds) (1995) *The Culture of Long Term Care: Nursing Home Ethnography.* London: Bergin and Garvey.

Hepworth, M. (1991) 'Positive ageing and the mask of age.' *Journal of Educational Gerontology 6,* 2, 93–101.

Hepworth, M. (2000) *Stories of Ageing.* Buckingham: Open University Press.

Hockey, J. and James, A. (1993) *Growing Up and Growing Old: Ageing and Dependency in the Life Course.* London: Sage.

Holstein, J.A. and Gubrium, J.F. (2000) *The Self We Live By: Narrative Identity in a Postmodern World.* New York: Oxford University Press.

Ignatieff, M. (1994) *Scar Tissue.* London: Vintage.

Kitwood, T. (1997) *Dementia Reconsidered: The Person Comes First.* Buckingham: Open University Press.

Lee-Treweek, G. (1998) 'Bedroom abuse: the hidden work in a nursing home.' In M. Allot and M. Robb (eds) *Understanding Health and Social Care.* London: Sage.

Lyman, K.A. (1989) 'Bringing the social back in: a critique of the bio-medicalisation of dementia.' *The Gerontologist 29*, 5, 597–604.

Lyman, K.A. (1993) *Day In, Day Out with Alzheimer's: Stress in Caregiving Relationships.* Philadelphia: Temple.

Manthorpe, J. (1996) 'Dementia in contemporary fiction: from outside looking in…' *Journal of Dementia Care 4*, 2, 27–29.

Manthorpe, J. (2000) 'Dementia in contemporary fiction and biography.' *Journal of Dementia Care 83*, 35–37.

McColgan, G., Valentine, J. and Downs, M. (2000) 'Concluding narratives of a career with dementia: accounts of Iris Murdoch at her death.' *Ageing and Society 20*, 1, 97–109.

McGowin, D.F. (1993) *Living in the Labyrinth: A Personal Journey through the Maze of Alzheimer's.* San Francisco: Elder.

Post, S.G. (1995) *The Moral Challenge of Alzheimer Disease.* Baltimore and London: Johns Hopkins University Press.

Rose, L. (1996) *Show Me the Way to Go Home.* San Francisco: Elder.

Sabat, S.R. (1994) 'Excess disability and malignant social psychology: a case study of Alzheimer's Disease.' *Journal of Community and Applied Social Psychology 4*, 157–166.

Sacks, H., Schegloff, E.A. and Jefferson, G. (1974) 'A simplest systematics for the organization of turn-taking for conversation.' *Language 50*, 4, 1, 696–735.

Savishinsky, J.S. (1991) *The Ends of Time: Life and Work in a Nursing Home.* London: Bergin and Garvey.

Schegloff, E.A. and Sacks, H. (1973) 'Opening up closings.' *Semiotica VIII*, 4, 289–327.

Strauss, A. (1997) *Mirrors and Masks: The Search for Identity.* New Brunswick and London: Transaction Publishers.

Wark Clements (Producers) (2003) 'Kirsty meets Kate and Rikki Fulton.' In series *Lives Less Ordinary.* BBC Scotland, transmitted 3 March.

CHAPTER 12

Reaching Out with the Arts: Meeting with the Person with Dementia

Claire Craig
Postscript by John Killick

I have arrived at the hospital to begin my placement. I will be here for ten weeks. It is a large cavernous building. Imposing. Impersonal. My supervisor has given me a tour of the wards and finally takes me to Ward Eight, the ward for people with dementia. Immediately as we walk through the doors I am struck by the smell of stale urine. It feels unwelcoming. There is little decoration except for a sign which tells visitors that drinks of coffee are 15p a cup.

My supervisor whisks me into the main sitting room. The staff are congregated around the television, drinking coffee and chatting, while yards away people with dementia are sitting. One gentleman is lying on the floor; another lady is polishing using a piece of tissue. One person is sitting in a chair so low to the ground that he is unable to stand. Ever so often I see him place his hands on the chair arms, push himself up and then drop back down again. It is noisy and chaotic. A lady approaches and pleads with me to take her home, pulling on my arm. Swiftly a nurse intercepts, leading her away to a chair.

The staff on the ward are friendly, interested and I tell them that I would like to spend time here and wonder what input the occupational therapist might have. They seem thrilled but then my supervisor interrupts. She does not envisage my spending large amounts of time here. She tells me that we will assess the 'more able' individuals and those with the highest level of cognitive functioning will be able to attend groups in the department. These individuals are my priority as there is very little that we can offer the individuals with greatest need, no evidence of therapeutic benefits. She is disapproving of my 'notion' of the potential of the arts and creativity.

This is the reality of marginalisation. It is a bleak image but one I believe that is not unique. I have observed many similar situations during my own work as an occupational therapist in the care environments where people with dementia live. John Killick has also written of deep, meaningful conversations with individuals who have been dismissed by staff and clinicians as 'having nothing important to say' (Killick 1997). These are worrying descriptions in the age of the 'new culture of dementia care' (Kitwood 1995). However, this chapter will explore:

- the potential of creativity in providing a way forward
- how the marginalisation of people with dementia can be countered through the arts
- what these opportunities may be and who should lead them.

Throughout this chapter I hope to illustrate that it is no longer tenable to consider the arts as a luxury. Their role in providing a medium for communication, self-expression and the continual reinforcement of identity means that they are in fact a necessity and should therefore be seen in the widest context, not something separate but as part of the everyday environments in which people with dementia live.

We listen to and reflect on the stories that people with dementia tell and we learn that the lived experience of dementia for many individuals is one of denied opportunity, environmental constraints, changing roles, social isolation and the stripping away of possessions or belongings. It is the reality of wearing clothes that aren't your own, not being able to express yourself, to really express your anger or frustration or sadness without questions regarding medication. The 'old culture of dementia care' described dementia as being an assault on identity. I would argue that on many occasions this 'assault' is more the consequence of our struggle to communicate and to find a different language in order to connect with the person. The expectation is that the person with dementia will meet with us on our terms using language that is familiar. This is no longer acceptable. People with dementia show us that we must find new ways of communicating.

We listen to other voices and realise that we must also re-examine the physical and social environments where many individuals with dementia live and ask whether the setting supports or denies personhood. For example we must look again at the bed bays, which have become people's homes, and ask whether it is possible to gain a sense of who someone is from the environment which supports and which holds them or whether this in itself contributes to the insidious process of depersonalisation, which can often occur.

For instance Jack, who has been an athlete, known throughout the county for his prowess and who has represented his region at his sport, lies in a sterile bed bay. This place that has been his home for the last 10, 15 years bears not a single object, possession or photograph that would indicate anything of who he is, what is important to him, where he has travelled. There is not a single clue to indicate who his family are or to provide an introduction to his vast circle of friends. The room is stripped of all identity with its white walls, white linen and a single bedside cabinet. Only his name and the name of his consultant, handwritten on a wipeable board above his bed, provide an indication of who this gentleman is. Jack's physical needs make it difficult for him to mobilise. He doesn't verbally communicate so it is impossible to let the steady stream of bank staff and temporary carers know anything about him. Many have read the notes, which speak of medication, of the regularity of his bowel movements, of the importance of turning him every few hours to prevent the development of pressure sores. There isn't a mention in these notes of what he holds as being important, about his wife, his interests, his love of jazz music, his enjoyment of being with and of seeing his grandchildren.

I watch the temporary care staff working with him and observe them speaking over this gentleman as they turn and move him in bed. Their conversation focuses on what they have been doing the evening before, what to wear tonight and the latest gossip on 'Coronation Street'. Not a single attempt is made to speak to Jack, to address him directly. He has become a body to be moved and fed and toileted. I speak with the staff afterwards and they tell me that they literally don't know what to say to him. How could they, when they don't know who he is? All they see is a person who lies in bed day after day not moving, not speaking. One of the staff speaks of feeling a little 'frightened'; they describe how uncomfortable the silence is and their feelings of embarrassment when conversation is not responded to.

I spend time with Jack and his family. His wife is thrilled when I ask her to bring in precious photographs of their wedding day, of their first child's christening, of a family get together with Jack sat at the head of the table. I make high quality copies of the images and discover that Jack is able to express preferences through eye pointing. We work together and he chooses images to frame. We spend time sitting, listening to jazz music as I build the frames. At times he lies with his eyes closed, moving to the music; at others he is very much involved in the decoration of the frames, in the sponging of the paint. The images are mounted and placed where he can see them. Other staff comment and I hear them speaking to Jack, talking about the images, what they can see. Conversation. The recognition of the person behind the label of the illness.

We provide more appropriate seating so that Jack is able to sit out of bed at certain times of the day. I find a range of musical instruments hidden away in the occupational therapy cupboard. Jack minutely taps out a beat. I mirror this back to him. The movements over time become more confident. There are clues that he is beginning to recognise who I am, to initiate requests. For instance now when I walk into the bed bay he turns his whole body to look at the CD player and I instinctively ask, 'Music, Jack?' A nod of the head. Sometimes he points his finger at an image. 'Would you like to look at the photograph, Jack?' No response. 'Oh, are you asking whether Margaret is coming in today?' Eye contact. 'Yes she is.' A tiny movement of the lips as though a smile.

These snippets of Jack's story begin to highlight the central role that the arts can play in redressing the imbalances of dementia in overcoming the marginalisation that many individuals face. Their emphasis on individuality, expression, on the uniqueness of being, can help the person to begin to re-establish a sense of self, to rebuild identity. Painting, music, writing, art, dance, photography, drama can provide those all-important bridges, those meeting places where our world and the world of the person overlap, where feelings and emotions can be expressed and communication at the deepest level can occur using a language that is not necessarily dependent upon words.

If this is the way forward then we must dismiss the old notions that the arts are exclusive, confined only to individuals with higher levels of cognitive functioning. We must also revisit ideas that the arts are prescriptive, judged only on aesthetic merit, on an end result. The arts are for everyone and by their very nature are all encompassing. Therefore the sensory and expressive qualities of the media that are used, the process of engagement, the relationship between artist, material and onlooker are all key and should not be ignored. The arts are about meaningful engagement but they are about so much more than the 'filling of time' – something that Suzanne Peloquin expresses very clearly when she writes:

> The image of someone in the act of making is one in which human being (character, heart spirit) flows into human doing. The difference between doing and making is one of substance rather than semantic. Making suggests a creation. (Peloquin 1997, pp.167–8)

The arts present many possibilities for people with dementia. These include the following.

Opportunities for enjoyment

The arts can provide opportunities for social interaction, for fun, the sharing of experiences, engaging the senses. A person may experience pleasure from completing the activity itself. As one gentleman with dementia declared after a paper marbling session: 'It's not just good. It's marvellous.'

On many occasions it is through the sharing of the activity, of developing relationship, reflected in the comments of Dorothy after she had made her first piece of handmade felt: 'I do hope that we can do that tomorrow because you've right cheered me up.'

Expression of emotions

Music, art, dance, poetry can all provide powerful vehicles for the expression of emotions. Music in particular has the ability to impact on mood, tapping into deep memories. An Irish jig, an uplifting melody can transform the atmosphere. There have been wonderful moments when a person, seemingly 'locked' into themselves, has started to move in response to a piece of music. As Sandy Crichton writes,

> Music plays an invigorating role, like a co-leader in a movement session. Live music is wonderful to move to… Taped music can transform the atmosphere, frame the dancing. Singing, dancing and music-making go alongside each other, one flowing into the other. (Crichton 1997, p.17)

Painting activities similarly have the potential to provide opportunities for self-expression. On many occasions the materials or the image has provided the person with the necessary space to speak about deep emotions. Individuals have communicated through the work or the materials to express fears, worries, feelings. For instance during a session using decoupage one lady, rejecting flowers and animals to adorn her box, chose instead a small girl dressed in Victorian costume. She placed the picture on the inside of the box and quickly closed the lid. Quite unprompted she told me, 'She feels very alone and frightened. What do you make of that?' I told her that it must be difficult and she nodded her head slowly and said, 'Yes I really miss my sister. I wish she could be here for me to talk to' (Craig 2001, p.36).

Gaining a sense of control

Arts sessions provide vital opportunities for the person to exercise skills in choice and decision making and in the expression of preferences. This can occur at a number of levels. For instance Sterritt and Pokorny (1994) have described how arts activities provided the means by which individuals attending a day centre were able to gain feelings of control. Similarly Foster and McMorland (1993) have described how artwork formed the vehicle for individuals with dementia to gain a sense of mastery over the environment in which they were living.

Reminiscence

One gentleman, Arthur, shared the following description of an early memory of art during a creative session:

> I remember being young. We'd use a toothbrush, make a square and flick the paint. It was all a bit messy really. Never mind. I'm quite impressed by this though. I didn't have time to look at what came out.

The arts can provide wonderful opportunities for the sharing of memories. For instance, Judith Perry (1997) has described her work with people with dementia and how creative work with textiles formed a powerful vehicle for reminiscence and the celebration of individuals' life stories.

Reinforcing identity

Karen Jarvis writes:

> One theme has emerged from all the collage work I have undertaken with clients and that is the importance of identity. Let them tell us, or show us, perhaps through collage, who they are. (Jarvis 1998, p.8)

Framed photographs, pieces of artwork, textiles decorating the place where the person lives can help to reinforce a person's sense of individuality and make personal space personal. As a result it can become possible to gain a sense of who someone is from the place in which they live.

Self-esteem

The arts provide opportunities for individuals to gain a sense of mastery or achievement. Emma Snelling, Mike Bender and Denise Gregson have written of the role of the arts in restoring the give and take in a relationship. They describe a series of arts sessions where people with dementia were given the opportunity to create gifts for families and for friends. They write of the experience:

> For the clients, this group proved to be a positive and productive experience for those participating in the group, and for the relatives who received the gifts... The group was emotionally powerful for both the members and their relatives. (Snelling *et al.* 2000, p.20)

As a stimulus for imagination and communication

The following was spoken by Mary, in response to a piece of paper that she had marbled. It is written down exactly as she described it using her words.

> How beautiful it is.
> You can see all sorts of pictures in it.
> A man's face, all cross and angry.
>
> A jellyfish with its legs tangled up.
> The side of a map,
> Look where the water goes in.
>
> That part's like a trumpet,
> All bright and shiny.
> Ah look at the red room
>
> Champagne and rubies.
> But this one is my favourite.
> It's electoplasm.
>
> (Craig 2003, pp.45–6, reproduced with kind permission from
> Dementia Services Development Centre, University of Stirling)

Arts sessions provide spaces where people with dementia can express themselves imaginatively in this way. On many occasions the person may not use words at all. For instance Sandy Crichton in her work using Jabadao, with its focus on communication through movement, writes that Jabadao:

offers a means of rich communication without the necessity of speech: an avenue of direct communication through movement. When words no longer flow easily, or become unreliable and treacherous, this is painful for all concerned. Using movement to communicate can be a relief and release. (Crichton 1997, p.16)

Challenging preconceptions

The arts often challenge us to revisit our preconceptions about who a person with dementia is. Many times when I have been sitting in the office writing notes I have overheard conversations relating to individual pieces of work produced by the person with dementia. 'Mr A, president of where? Well who'd have thought it.'

Similarly in describing an arts project with people with dementia Helen Nairn writes:

> Although we had realised that our residents had untapped potential, we still found ourselves amazed at the response some of the activities brought. Several times we excitedly recounted stories to each other about what residents had done. (Nairn 1995, p.16)

Increasing feelings of well-being

Paul Batson writes of his work using drama with people with dementia:

> As people with dementia become increasingly withdrawn the use of drama can provide another means of stimulation that enables them to relate with others and experience increased moments of well being. (Batson 1998, p.21)

These are just a few examples but more importantly people with dementia are telling us the importance of the arts in the context of their lives. James McKillop writes:

> ...being told that I had dementia led to a door reopening after a difficult time in my life. New challenges, new friendships. I wanted to raise awareness about dementia and show that people with dementia can relearn forgotten skills as well as learn something new. (McKillop 2002, p.7)

Another lady told John Killick, 'The arts, is all that's left. Give them to us!!' (Killick 2002, p.26).

There is a sense of urgency in these words, which we cannot afford to ignore. The arts challenge us. They ask that we look again from a different perspective, to spend time listening and revisiting our beliefs about who someone with dementia is. I have at times in my own work experienced a jarring of my sensibilities when I have looked at the marks that a person has made, reflected on the words that someone has spoken, an expressive movement, a response, and I have realised that I have been literally blinded by the label of dementia. I have failed to look, to really look beyond the surface, to ask probing questions of the information, the clinical terms and to see that there is a person at the heart.

We may have to revisit preconceptions about the skills that a person with dementia has or is able to develop. Often there is the notion that the cognitive changes that occur affect an individual's ability to abstract or to learn new information. Yet I have observed a person who has significant cognitive difficulties engage in complex tasks and learn new skills, for instance in the making of handmade felt or watercolour painting. I am not alone in these observations. Miller (2001) is involved in ongoing research with people with frontotemporal dementia and findings to date suggest that a number of individuals were able to continue practising art forms successfully after the onset of the condition while others developed new aptitudes and reached a high level of proficiency in their chosen medium.

Perhaps one of the most beautiful published collections of artwork by people with dementia reflecting the scope of this new learning is in the *Memories in the Making* book by Selly Jenny (Jenny and Oropeza 1993) which catalogues the works produced in a programme of creative art sessions with individuals with Alzheimer's disease. These skills are not confined to art and painting. The sculptures of Christophe Grillet in Cambridge again reflect the extent to which new, exceptionally complex skills can be developed. It is essential that we do not underestimate an individual's potential for creativity. I remember all too clearly watching a lady, who had been dismissed by many as having too great a level of need to benefit from arts sessions, pick up a ball of discarded wool and begin to finger knit (Craig 2001, p.4).

On many occasions dementia has led a person with whom I have been working to re-discover lost skills or there has been a flowering of creativity. This seems ironic when so much emphasis is placed on the 'losses' which dementia encapsulates. Yet frequently as these 'cognitive losses' increase I have observed a compensatory increase in other skills that the person possesses, perhaps a reflection of the human need for maintaining a sense of connectedness with others.

John Killick has argued convincingly that while dementia attacks the 'logical powers of the brain it leaves many of the emotional capacities intact. As feeling persons, people with the condition have much to come to terms with, and the arts provide a variety of possibilities for self-expression' (Killick 2002, p.26). John's work has shown us the importance of recognising the qualities of the words that people with dementia use when he writes:

> The language used by people with dementia is a metaphorical one – where what they say often doesn't make sense in the usual literal way but has a poetic or symbolic meaning. People express themselves in a language nearer to poetry than they used to before. (Killick 1994, p.17)

If the arts are seen as a vehicle for communication perhaps we need also to understand the expressive quality of the materials used. Without this understanding, this experience would be the equivalent of learning a language from a book or a tape but never having the opportunity to speak it, or to listen to a description of a chocolate cake, to its flavours, without ever tasting it. Until you have savoured the bitterness of the chocolate or the lightness of the sponge perhaps it is not possible to grasp the true nature of its consistency, its taste, its flavour from either watching someone eat the cake or from listening to a description of it.

As an amateur painter I know only too well that until you have experienced the stickiness of acrylic paint, the fluidity of watercolour, the absorbency of the paper it is difficult to comprehend their potential strengths and limitations as a medium. You are effectively an onlooker and not a participant in the process. The strength of the arts is that they can work on so many different levels. Yet some of the most meaningful arts sessions I have experienced have been when I have sat alongside a person and engaged with the medium and the paper has formed the record of our dialogue. When colour and texture has been the language and the paper has formed the meeting place. The tone and the pressure of the marks have in fact been the expression of emotions. On many occasions I have not understood the exact nature of these but it has been sufficient to acknowledge their existence.

The following is a small extract from my own reflective journal of painting with a lady with dementia who lived in a residential care setting.

> The abstract image is tiny. Swirls of magenta and vermilion intermingled on the watercolour paper. Rich, delicate. It represents a meeting between Margaret and I. Each line has been considered. Initially the marks were faltering as she tried out the materials, gained a sense of the paint, exercised choice, selected the colours, mastered the brush. The final layers are richer, more definite, a tribute to her growing confidence. In the very early sessions she would watch as I sat during my break, with my scraps of watercolour

paper, making marks. Sometimes she would help me choose the colours, delighting in this new-found control in a world where she wasn't even given the choice over what she ate for lunch or when she ate it. In time I have discovered her wicked sense of humour, a real sense of fun which she expresses in so many ways – a huge splodge in the middle of an otherwise ordered piece. Her rebellion. Sometimes all I gain is a sense of her frustration as she scribbles over the paper with frantic marks. Fast pace, fast rhythm, intense, absorbed. On other occasions she is weary, tired, disinterested, making tiny faint marks which I mirror back to her on the paper.

I frame the image and watch Margaret (against my better judgement) offer it to a member of staff in the home. The staff look and ask what it is. I intercept and say 'it's an abstract' but I can see that they don't understand. 'I thought it was a flower' one of the carers replies, disappointed. This reflects so much of how they see her. All surface, never looking beyond. Nothing deeper.

The image is hung on a wall. I should feel pleased, it is a tribute to Margaret and her skills, but instead I feel vulnerable, relieved that I will be leaving soon to begin my training. After I have gone, the painting will be there as a concrete record for all to see of a journey that we have travelled together, the joys and frustrations that we have shared in trying to express ourselves through the language of the paint.

For Margaret and myself painting represented a space where we could be ourselves. It was a relationship of equals. When we were painting we were engaging at every level, including emotionally. It was at this level that the paints communicated most powerfully.

By their very nature, the arts raise many questions. For instance John Killick highlights the important question as to who should lead the activities: 'therapists or artists or enthusiasts or staff?' (Killick 2002, p.26). My reply to this is that we can all bring different things to the relationship. The therapist will have an awareness of the components of the activity, of the skills required to engage in the process and how the activity can be used and adapted for meaningful engagement so that the needs of the individual can be met. Artists will have more of an instinctive understanding of the qualities of the materials themselves, of the language of art and the struggles that may be faced when working with the creative media, whether it is words, images, marks, music, movement, drama, dance. Enthusiasts will by definition bring an excitement, an energy, a playfulness to the process. I believe too that carers have a key role to play. The wealth of experience, knowledge and deep emotion that a carer possesses means that the arts could provide the means by which those all-important connections can be established and re-established. The under-standing and sensitivity that spouses, children, grandchildren, friends bring to this relationship cannot be rivalled.

Importantly we need to begin to share ideas and ways of working. If marginalisation is to be overcome then we cannot afford to be precious with the skills that we possess. We need to examine the artistic media that we use and ensure that it is of the highest quality so that the individual is supported and not hindered by the materials themselves. Equally the arts and creativity cannot be confined to specially designated sessions, separate from the day-to-day routines and the fabric of places where people live. As Dawn Brooker states:

> Therapeutic activities can no longer be seen as something that are 'done to' people with dementia according to a timetable drawn up by busy professionals working Monday to Friday, 9am to 5pm. We have moved into an era now where it is seen as desirable that the whole environment (social, psychological and physical) is geared up to the promotion of optimal well-being. (Brooker 2001, p.159)

Perhaps most challenging of all we should sit back and trust the process itself. We must not be frightened to explore unfamiliar territory. At times there will not be a clear scientific explanation to help us understand what is happening and we will instead be required to trust what we are seeing and experiencing in our interactions. This may feel uncomfortable at times. However, I believe that we can learn much from spending time exploring the materials and from reflecting on their expressive qualities and on our own attitudes towards them. The arts offer such potential in reaching out to meet with the person, to provide a medium for communication, a source of stimulation, a means to restore and reinforce identity, and to ignore them would be to deny the person with dementia. Finally:

> The placement has come to an end. Ten weeks have flown by. I feel that I have hardly scratched the surface but there have been minute shifts such as the way that the chairs are arranged, the introduction of sessions on the ward. Tiny battles have been won. Images now adorn the walls. Marbled paper created by individuals on the ward, images of landscapes chosen by Frank and Ernest. I am sitting on Ward Eight. The staff are still congregated in a corner of the room but they are open, smiling, interested. The television isn't on and there is music playing in the background. Alice and John are swaying in time to the melody; Ernest has already taken me for a spin around an imaginary dance floor. It is a starting point but there is a sense of change and I know that the arts are at last beginning to work their magic.

Postscript by John Killick

Clare has made the case eloquently for the arts to percolate throughout dementia care, refreshing areas which have hitherto been neglected. Do we have to wait for this process to take effect, the slow drip of good practice to gradually change attitudes and create an ambience in which creativity is encouraged and valued? Is there anything we can do to hasten that process?

Well, first of all the arts in healthcare is a national movement which in Britain is growing apace. Conferences are now being held in which practitioners gather to share experiences and to hear of new developments. Organisations are being set up to get the arts put on the agenda in medical and care settings ('National Network for the Arts in Health'); to underline the therapeutic nature of what the arts can offer ('Arts Therapists Working with Older People'); and to stress the positive effects of activity when set against the impoverished environments where physical well-being alone is promoted ('National Association of Providers of Activities'). We must see that the needs of people with dementia are given prominence in each forum.

Second, we must combat the paternalism which so regularly and depressingly raises its head when artworks are created by people with dementia. The grudging acknowledgement that something has been brought into existence is a long way from the heartfelt endorsement of the true quality of achievement that is called for. So often the attitude that lies behind people's reactions is similar to that of Dr Johnson when he remarked of women attempting to preach: 'It is not done well, but you are surprised to find it done at all.' Or the infantilisation of people with the condition, which judges any achievement by the standard of an untutored child, when so manifestly the expressive content is that of someone with a whole lifetime of experience behind them. We must counter this disempowerment wherever it occurs; it is cousin to the 'personal detractions' of Bradford Dementia Group's Dementia Care Mapping method (1997). Paintings, poems, sculptures, photographs etc. by people with dementia can be of a standard comparable with the best of those produced by people without the condition, and we do their creators a grave disservice by putting them in an enclave labelled 'dementia', and thereby ensuring their devaluation.

This leads directly on to my third proposal for moving the arts and dementia care forward. There needs to be training for staff in every kind of setting so that they welcome interventions of this kind, appreciate the importance of process in this kind of work, and give an appropriate welcome to any outcomes which emerge from that process. Parallel to this, artists who have not worked in this field before could benefit from guidance on what to expect from interactions with people with dementia, as communication is a vital aspect of the work and lack of appreciation of this can easily lead to failure.

Lastly, a proposal to break down the barriers between the generations. Although there are younger people with dementia, it is predominantly found in old age, and this group suffers a double disadvantage: the low esteem in which older people are held, and the mixture of fear and incomprehension which often greets people with the condition. A way of countering this is to deliberately mix the generations up. There is often a disinhibited childlikeness shown by people with dementia which makes integrating them with children an attractive and productive proposition. 'Magic Me' is an organisation in Britain which has been particularly successful in mounting projects of this kind, and at Stirling University we hope to do more of the same, and to link this work with proper training courses for artists and staff.

It is the nature of marginalisation that it is unlikely to go away unless we adopt a proactive stance. It is the nature of dementia that those with the condition find it difficult to mount a consistent and coherent strategy to counter marginalisation. It is the nature of the arts that they can help to create a climate in which such imaginative leaps become a possibility. Therefore we must harness them in our attempt to make greater integration in society a reality.

References

Batson, P. (1998) 'Drama as therapy: bringing memories to life.' *Journal of Dementia Care* July/August, 19–21.

Bradford Dementia Group (1997) *Evaluating Dementia Care: The DCM Method.* Bradford: University of Bradford.

Brooker, D. (2001) 'Therapeutic activity.' In C. Cantley (ed) *A Handbook of Dementia Care.* Buckingham: Open University Press.

Craig, C. (2001) *Celebrating the Person: A Practical Approach to Art Activities.* Stirling: Dementia Services Development Centre, Stirling University.

Craig, C. (2003) *Meaningful Making: A Practice Guide for Occupational Therapy Staff.* Stirling: Dementia Services Development Centre. Stirling University.

Crichton, S. (1997) 'Moving is the language I use. Communication is my goal.' *Journal of Dementia Care*, November/December, 16–17.

Foster, K. and McMorland, A. (1993) *Art Prints in Residential Homes.* Stirling: Dementia Services Development Centre, Stirling University.

Jarvis, K. (1998) 'Recovering a lost sense of identity.' *Journal of Dementia Care* 6, 3, 7–8.

Jenny, S. and Oropeza, M. (1993) *Memories in the Making – A Programme of Creative Art Expression for Alzheimer Patients.* California: Alzheimer's Association of Orange County.

Killick, J. (1994) 'There's so much to hear when you stop and listen to individual voices.' *Journal of Dementia Care 2*, 5, 16–17.

Killick, J. (1997) 'Communication: a matter of life and death of the mind.' *Journal of Dementia Care*, September/October, 14–16.

Killick, J. (2002) 'Holding a rainbow in our hands: creativity in dementia.' In *Dementia: An Inclusive Future?* Symposium abstracts. Stirling: Dementia Services Development Centre, Stirling University.

Kitwood, T. (1995) *The New Culture of Dementia Care*. London: Hawker Publications.

McKillop, J. (2002) *Creativity in Dementia Care Calendar 2003*. London: Hawker Publications.

Miller, B. (2001) 'Functional correlates of musical and visual ability in frontotemporal dementia.' *British Journal of Psychiatry 176*, 458–463.

Nairn, H. (1995) 'Discover the difference activities can make.' *Journal of Dementia Care*, January/February, 16–18.

Peloquin, S.M. (1997) 'The spiritual depth of occupation: making worlds and making lives.' *American Journal of Occupational Therapy 51*, 3, 167–168.

Perry, J. (1997) 'The rich texture of memories.' *Journal of Dementia Care 5*, 4, 16–17.

Snelling, E., Bender, M. and Gregson, D. (2000) 'Restoring the give and take in a relationship.' *Journal of Dementia Care 8*, 1, 18–19.

Sterritt, P.F. and Pokorny, M.E. (1994) 'Art activities for patients with Alzheimer's and related disorders.' *Geriatric Nursing 15*, 3, 155–159.

PART 5

Future Directions

CHAPTER 13

Medical Perspectives

Michael Bradbury, Clive Ballard and Andrew Fairbairn

Introduction

This brief chapter will attempt to identify medical aspects of dementia where research attention has not been focused for some time. This is not to recognise the immense contribution the biomedical research in the field of dementia has made over the last 30 years. During that time we have gone from a concept of the inevitability of senility through to sophisticated scientific research including the latest neuropathological neurochemical and genetic investigations of the brain. It may be that certain medical aspects of the illness of a dementia have simply had the spotlight moved off them but may now deserve to be revisited as sophisticated new techniques become available, not least MRI scanning and SPECT scanning.

The relationship between early dementia and depression

There is a complex relationship between depression and the onset of dementia and also the co-morbidity of depression with early dementia. It is the author's personal view that modern research-driven classification systems such as DSM IV R (American Psychiatric Association 1994) in turn create limitations in phenomenological research, as there is a tendency to force diagnosis into boxes and perhaps miss broader opportunities to learn from syndromes.

It has been known for some time that, on a population not individual level, poor prognosis in depression in older people may be a prodrome of dementia.

A consistent view of depression in early dementia is also problematic. Is this an insightful reaction to a distressing disease? Is it a biologically based depression secondary to the biochemical changes of dementia?

O'Brien speculates on a 'cortisol theory' of depression and dementia where stress leads to hypercholesterolaemia and in turn leads on to hippocampal brain atrophy (O'Brien *et al.* 1994, pp.633–40). Another fashionable concept is that of 'vascular depression' (Alexopoulos *et al.* 1997, pp.915–22) – in essence, a group of elderly individuals suffering from depression with poor prognosis show increased evidence of white matter changes. This is presumed to be evidence of small vessel disease; that is, a vascular basis for a depression.

Finally, returning to the evidence that poor prognosis of depression may be a hint that the individual is going to develop a dementia, I am not aware of any work which attempts to correlate disease progression – for example, is a relatively rapid dementia associated with previous onset of depression? – yet this could be an important diagnostic marker.

Insight

A few years ago one of the authors discussed insight in dementia from the perspective of a practising clinician who was interested but ignorant about the concept of insight in dementia (Fairbairn 1997, pp.13–17). In the presentation that this chapter builds on, we have asked a number of questions:

1.   If insight is subjective, is it possible to test objectively?

2.   Is insight of any significance in disease progression?

3.   Is it related to premorbid factors such as intelligence?

It gradually became obvious that the world had moved on! Colleagues such as Linda Clare have done considerable work in this field in the last few years and their work is covered in a later chapter in which some of our questions are answered.

Capacity issues

The issue of mental capacity in dementia, in particular, has had increased attention since the Bournewood Judgement in the House of Lords. Briefly, a lower court had found that if an individual did not have capacity to object to an informal admission then they had to be detained under the Mental Health

Act in order to give them the protection of that Act. The House of Lords' judgement overturned this finding but there are suspicions that this might have been done for pragmatic, resource-driven reasons in that it is possible that the majority of people with dementia would then have potentially been subject to the Mental Health Act with all the resource consequences of that. The current situation is therefore that informal admission of a patient with dementia and lacking capacity can be justified on a duty of care basis by the doctor but, of course, this leaves the patient with no system to look after his/her best interests.

The Lord Chancellor's Office, after a long period of gestation, have finally resurrected proposals for mental incapacity legislation, building on the *Who Decides?* document of 1995 (Lord Chancellor's Department 1995). Current controversies in relation to a revised English Mental Health Act look as if they will unfortunately be unaffected by the incapacity proposals. In Scotland, the whole premise of their Mental Health Act legislation, is based on an initial clinical judgement of capacity.

Finally, in this section, one of the tragedies of loss of capacity in dementia is that the individual is unable to contribute to complex decisions in relation to end of life issues. Advance directives might address this but there is believed to be little enthusiasm to formalise advance directives in future incapacity legislation.

Dementia as a systemic disease

The old descriptive textbooks of psychiatry such as Slater and Roth (1969) referred to dementia as a 'wasting' disease. In other words, there was a systemic effect from brain failure, possibly analogous to disuse atrophy in a stroke patient. It is interesting that in the chapters on dementia in the latest *Psychiatry in the Elderly* textbook (Jacoby and Oppenheimer 2002, 3rd edition) there is absolutely no reference to systemic aspects of dementia. In other words, we seem to be brilliantly concentrating on the brain but losing sight of the rest of the body!

The systemic impact of dementia could be relevant because, for example, significant weight loss directly attributable to a dementia could be a poor prognostic indicator.

The cause of death in dementia, that is Category 1 on the death certificate, is usually the terminal event and this is typically bronchopneumonia. Nevertheless, we are less than sure of the impact of the dementia on the cause of death. With a vascular dementia, it can be presumed that a further stroke might lead to death, but with Alzheimer's disease, the more severe the cognitive impairment, the more close to death is the patient, but there is certainly no simple predictability about this. The ability to improve prognosis in dementia, especially at the severe end of the spectrum, would be helpful for planning compassionate terminal care and for assisting relatives in their grieving process.

Vascular lesions and dementia

One of the best examples of the interface of physical disorders and dementia is the role of vascular disease and vascular risk factors in the development of progressive cognitive decline. Vascular dementia (VaD) itself is defined as a clinical syndrome of acquired clinical impairment resulting from brain injury due to cerebrovascular disorder (Tatemichi *et al.* 1994). The estimated lifetime risk of developing VaD is 35 per cent in men and 19 per cent in women (Hagnell *et al.* 1992). Furthermore, 20 per cent of patients have dementia in the aftermath of a stroke (Nyenhuis and Gorelick 1998), with 30 per cent of these patients developing dementia within three months (Jorm 1990). There is an elevated risk of incident dementia that lasts for at least five years (Tatemichi *et al.* 1994; Desmond *et al.* 2000).

The NINCDS AIRENS criteria (Roman *et al.* 1993) describe a number of different categories of VaD incorporating multi-infarct dementia, strategic single infarct dementia, extensive white matter disease, hypoperfusion and haemorrhagic dementia. These subdivisions, based around the NINCDS AIRENS framework, are described in Box 13.1.

The mechanisms by which these types of cerebrovascular pathology lead to dementia are unclear. The volume of cerebral infarct is clearly an important determinate of cognitive impairment, with all patients experiencing dementia having infarct volumes exceeding 50 ml (Brun 1994). Other vascular factors are also contributory; illustrating this, Esiri, Wilcock and Morris (1997) reported that microvascular disease rather than macroscopic infarction was the main association of dementia in patients with cerebrovascular disease.

Vascular lesions are also important in Alzheimer's disease (AD). For example, the incidence of AD in stroke patients is nine times higher than the general population and AD is three times more likely to occur following a stroke or a TIA (transient ischaemic attack) (Kokman *et al.* 1996). In addition, the overlap of cerebrovascular and neurodegenerative pathologies (Snowden *et al.* 1997) or concurrent cholinergic deficits (Perry *et al.* 1978) are likely to be important.

Box 13.1 The **NINCDS AIRENS** criteria for VaD

1. Multi-infarct dementia involves multiple large complete infarcts usually from large vessel occlusions involving cortical and sub-cortical areas resulting in a clinical syndrome of dementia.

2. Strategic single infarct dementia is due to small localised ischemic damage occurring in cortical and sub-cortical areas of the brain that result in specific clinical syndromes. For example infarcts to the angular gyrus result in the onset of fluent aphasis, alexia with agraphia, memory disturbance, spatial disorientation and constructional disturbances.

3. Small vessel disease or microvascular disease results from lesions that occur in either cortical or sub-cortical areas of the brain and often involve white matter. The lesions result in an occlusion of a single arteriolar or arterial lumen that leads to complete lacunar infarct. Critical stenosis of multiple small vessels can also occur, resulting in hypoperfusion and complete infarcts.

4. White matter disease or leukoaraiosis is frequently noted on structural brain imaging. The frequency of white matter disease is found to rise steadily with age. It has been found to be associated with hypertension, cigarette smoking, low plasma vitamin E, lacunar infarcts, low education, and hypoxic-ischemic disorders (Gorelick et al. 1999).

5. Hypoperfusion results from a global brain ischaemia secondary to cardiac arrest or profound hypertension, or from restricted ischaemia that has occurred in the border zones between two main arterial territories. Hemorrhagic dementia occurs due to chronic subdural hematoma, sequelae of subarachnoid hemorrhage, and a cerebral hematoma, and is often associated with amyloid angiopathy.

Neuropathological data indicates that AD and vascular lesions often co-exist (Del Ser *et al.* 1990; Ince *et al.* 1995; Jellinger *et al.* 1990; Victoroff *et al.* 1995), with 60 to 90 per cent of AD cases exhibiting cerebrovascular pathology. Autopsy studies have also found evidence of cerebral infarction in at least 35 per cent of AD patients (Olichney *et al.* 1995; Premkumar *et al.* 1996). Evidence shows that the clinical impact of concurrent neurodegenerative lesions is additive, with vascular lesions worsening the level of deficits and reducing the threshold of AD pathology necessary for the clinical presentation of dementia (Snowden *et al.* 1997).

Vascular dementia

Heart disease

A variety of aspects of heart disease are clearly related to cognitive function and dementia. For example, cardiac arrest (Reich *et al.* 1983), chronic heart disease (Arboix, Marti-Vilata and Garcia 1990; Barclay *et al.* 1988), myocardial infarction (Legault, Joffe and Armstrong 1992) and atrial fibrillation (Murgatroyd and Camm 1993) are all associated with cognitive impairment in older people. Women with a history of myocardial infarction are three times more likely than men to develop dementia and are five times more likely to develop dementia, especially AD, when compared to individuals with no history of myocardial infarction (Aronson *et al.* 1990). Atrial fibrillation increases the risk of dementia by two-fold especially in women and patients over the age of 75 (Ott *et al.* 1997), possibly because of reduced cardiac output leading to cerebral under-perfusion with related hypoxic brain damage and cognitive decline (Hachinski, Potter and Merskey 1987; Ylikoski *et al.* 1995). At least 15 per cent of patients with atrial fibrillation have silent infarctions (Ezekowitz *et al.* 1995; Feinberg *et al.* 1990), which have been shown to accelerate the progression of cognitive impairments in other patient groups (Ott *et al.* 1997).

Longitudinal studies have also demonstrated that cardiovascular diseases (Stewart *et al.* 1991) are predictors of cognitive impairment in the elderly population. The extent of cognitive impairment is often related to the severity of the cardiac disease. This is illustrated by studies examining the relationship between cognition and congestive cardiac failure, which have indicated an association between the degree of left ventricular dysfunction (Zuccala *et al.* 1997) and cognition. Reduced cardiac output and low systolic blood pressure have also been associated with white matter lesions on CT or MRI and dementia (Tavornen-Schroder *et al.* 1996). In addition to the relationship between cardiac disease and cognition, there is accumulating evidence of a link with pathological features of Alzheimer's disease. Cerebral amyloid plaques, which are characteristic of AD, have been found in non-demented patients with myocardial infarction (Sparks *et al.* 1990). Such plaques are distributed in a pattern similar to those found in Alzheimer's patients (Soneira and Scott 1998).

Hypertension

Hypertension is frequent in older people. Over a number of years, the elasticity of vessels is decreased, vascular resistance is increased and responsiveness to fluctuating changes in tissue demand is reduced (Barbro 1997; Farkas *et al.* 2000 & Meyer *et al.* 2000). Longitudinal studies that have investigated the effects of blood pressure on cognitive function have found an association between hypertension at midlife and impaired cognitive performance in later life (Carmelli *et al.* 1998) and an association between elevated blood pressure in midlife and the development of Alzheimer's disease (Kivipelto *et al.* 2000; Launer *et al.* 2000; Skoog *et al.* 1996). A study carried out by Fujishima and Tsuchihashi (1999) concluded that hypertension was also a risk factor for VaD. More recently the Canadian Study of Health and Aging (Herbert *et al.* 2000) established that hypertension was a significant risk factor for the development of VaD in females but not in males. In contrast Posner *et al.* (2002) reported that hypertension alone was not a risk factor for VaD; however, in comparison to controls there was a three-fold increase in the risk of dementia when hypertension was present in conjunction with heart disease. This risk was increased six-fold in hypertensive patients with diabetes. Low blood pressure has also been associated with cognitive impairment, AD and VaD (Breteler 1993; Guo *et al.* 1996; Hogan, Ebly and Rockwood 1997). Several epidemiological studies indicated that antihypertensive medication reduces the risk of dementia in patients with hypertension. Although the data is not entirely consistent there is preliminary evidence from placebo-controlled studies of antihypertensive treatment indicating the potential to prevent cognitive decline, particularly in higher risk groups. These studies are summarised in Table 13.1.

Diabetes

Type 2 diabetes mellitus is a common metabolic disorder that is most prevalent in middle-aged and elderly populations. It affects 8 to 10 per cent of people aged over 75 years and 14 per cent of those aged over 85 years (Croxon *et al.* 1991). Type 2 diabetes is associated with atherosclerosis of the cerebral arteries (Kameyama, Fushimi and Udaka 1994) and can lead to cerebrovascular changes that decrease cerebral blood flow (Mankovsky *et al.* 1992). Type 2 diabetes is a risk factor for lacunar and cerebral infarction (Lodder and Boiten 1993) and stroke (Stegmayr and Asplund 1995). Type 2 diabetes is also associated with white matter disease (Kinkel *et al.* 1985). A number of studies have indicated that patients with type 2 diabetes have an

Table 13.1 Effect of antihypertensive treatment on cognitive function and dementia

Key epidemiological studies	Sample size	Participants	Duration	Treatment	Reduction in BP	Impact on dementia or cognition
Murray et al. 2002	1900	Community-dwelling African Americans, 65	5 years	Various drugs as needed	Not reported	38% reduction in incident dementia (OR 0.62, 0.45–0.84)
Peila et al. 2001 (Honolulu-Asia aging study)	3605	Japanese-American men, mean age 53	26 years	Various drugs as needed	Not reported	Reduced risk of poor cognitive function (high systolic BP & ApoE4: OR 10.8 in untreated vs 1.9 in treated)
Guo et al. 2001 (Kungsholmen project)	985	Community-dwelling Swedish, 75	3 years	Various drugs as needed	Not reported	Reduced risk of dementia in those on antihypertensives at baseline (RR 0.6); effect more pronounced in ApoE carriers (RR 2.2 vs 0.9 on antihypertensives)
Forette et al. 1998 (Syst-Eur) Randomised controlled drug trials	2418	>60, Systolic hypertension	Median 2 years	Nitrendipine	8.3/3.8 mm Hg	50 per cent reduction in the incidence of dementia (7.7 to 3.8 cases per 1000 patient-years, p=0.05)

Study	N	Population	Duration	Intervention	BP reduction	Outcome
Forette *et al.* 2002 (Extended follow-up of Syst-Eur)	2902	60, Systolic hypertension	Median 3.9 years	Nitrendipine +- enalapril maleate +- hydrochlorothiazide	7.0/3.2 mm Hg	55% reduction in the risk of dementia (7.4 to 3.3 cases per 1000 patient-years, p=0.001)
Applegate *et al.* 1994 (systolic hypertension in the elderly)	2034	60, Systolic hypertension	5 years	Chlorthalidone		No significant impact of cognition or incident dementia
Prince *et al.* 1996 (MRC older people with HT)	2584	65–74, Systolic BP: 160–209 mm Hg	54 months	Atenolol, hydrochlorothiazide +- amiloride	17.1/- mm Hg	No significant impact on cognition or incident dementia
Bosch *et al.* 2002 (HOPE)	9297	>55, Left ventricular dysfunction	Mean 4.5 years	Ramipril, vitamin E	3.8/2.8 mm Hg	Significantly better outcome with respect to cognition and function
The PROGRESS Collaborative Group (2003)	6105	Mean age 64, Stroke or TIA with and without hypertension	4 years	Perindopril +- indapamide	9/4 mm Hg	Significant reduction in cognitive decline and incident dementia associated recurrent stroke
Lithell *et al.* 2003 (SCOPE)	4964	70–89, Systolic and/or diastolic hypertension	3.7 years	Candesartan (antihypertensive used in 84% of controls)	21.7/10.8 mm Hg	No difference on progression of cognitive impairment

elevated risk of developing dementia, both VaD and AD (Curb *et al.* 1999; Leibson *et al.* 1997; Ott *et al.* 1999; Yoshitake *et al.* 1995). For example, longitudinal studies have demonstrated that diabetes is associated with a higher incidence of VaD and AD (Kuusisto *et al.* 1997; Leisbon *et al.* 1997; Ott *et al.* 1999). Peila *et al.* (2002) estimated that type 2 diabetic patients had 1.5 (95% CI: 22–13.7) risk of developing dementia compared to non-diabetics, 2.3 (95% CI: 1.1–5.0) risk for the development of VaD and a 1.8 (95% CI: 1.1–2.9) risk for developing Alzheimer's disease which increased in subjects who carried the APOE $\in$ 4 allelle (5.5, 95% CI: 2.2–13.17).

In addition longitudinal studies have demonstrated an association between diabetes and cognitive deficits (Elias *et al.* 1997; Gregg *et al.* 2000; Strachan *et al.* 1997). For example women who had suffered with diabetes for more than 15 years had 57 to 114 per cent greater risk of major cognitive decline than women without diabetes (Gregg *et al.* 2000). The mechanisms are probably predominantly related to the severe microvascular disease, although intermittent hypoglycaemia may also be important. Hypoglycaemia has been found to disrupt cognitive functioning, with both diabetic and non-diabetic subjects showing performance deficits on test of memory, attention and executive function when glucose levels are reduced to 2.8 mmol/1 (Hoffman *et al.* 1989; Pramming *et al.* 1986).

Hence it has also been suggested that recurrent hypoglycaemia may have long-term adverse effects on intellect and cause dementia (Langan *et al.* 1991; Ryan *et al.* 1993). In addition, the risk of AD is slightly higher for patients with diabetes who use insulin rather than an oral hypoglycaemic agent (Luchsinger *et al.* 2001).

Delirium

Delirium is a common illness in frail older people (Levkoff *et al.* 1992; Rockwood 1994). Between 10 and 22 per cent of older patients are delirious on admission to hospital and 30 per cent or more of older medical patients develop delirium over the course of their hospital stay (Anthony *et al.* 1985; Inouye *et al.* 1993; Jitapunkel, Pillay and Ebrahim 1992; Johnson *et al.* 1990). People with dementia are at increased risk of delirium, but in addition delirium is associated with an increased risk of incident dementia (Koponen and Riekkinen 1983; Levkoff *et al.* 1992). In one study of 51 patients with delirium, dementia was diagnosed in 14 patients immediately after symptoms of delirium had subsided. An additional 14 patients developed dementia two years later. A total of 14 patients were diagnosed with AD or mixed dementia, 10 with VaD and two having dementia with Lewy bodies (Rahkonen *et al.* 2000). Rockwood *et al.* (1999) reported that 60 per cent of patients diagnosed with 'delirium – no dementia at baseline' went on to develop dementia within three years. There was a risk factor of 18.1 per cent for those with delirium compared to a 5.6 per cent risk for the controls without delirium. Further studies have also indicated that hospitalised patients with delirium and dementia experience a decline in cognition even after the delirium resolves (Fick and Foreman 2000).

Medical (Francis, Martin and Kapoor 1990; Inouye *et al.* 1993; Levkoff *et al.* 1992), surgical (Marcantonio *et al.* 1994) and psychiatric patients (Koponen and Riekkinen 1983) suffering with dementia have been found to be at high risk of developing delirium. Men are more at risk of developing delirium than women (Fisher and Flowerdew 1995; Williams-Russo *et al.* 1992). However, male gender may be a marker for alcohol abuse (Marcantonio *et al.* 1994) and alcoholism increases the risk of delirium three-fold (Elie *et al.* 1998). Depression also increases risk of delirium (Elie *et al.* 1998). Depression is associated with physical illness in the elderly, and elderly patients who are physically (Marcantonio *et al.* 1994), visually or hearing impaired are at risk of delirium (Elie *et al.* 1998). Patients suffering from previous stroke, structural brain abnormalities, brain cancer and cerebral metastasis (Rolfson *et al.* 1999) are also at risk. Other factors include bladder catheterisation, physical restraints (Inouye and Charpentier 1996; Werner *et al.* 1989), number of hospital procedures (Martin *et al.* 2000), quality of care (Inouye 1999), environment factors associated with hospital admissions and lack of activity and social interaction (Duppils and Wikbald 2001; Foreman 1989; Williams *et al.* 1985). Hence these are important considerations in the management of older people with or at risk of cognitive impairment, particularly as many cases can be prevented with simple interventions if those at risk are identified (Inouye 1999).

Anti-Alzheimer medication

The use of anti-Alzheimer medication in Alzheimer's disease is now reasonably well established and its use in dementia with Lewy bodies, although technically 'off-formulary', is also established clinical practice. What is less established but anecdotally intriguing is the use of anti-Alzheimer medication, that is cholinesterase inhibitors, as anti-psychotics. They are found to be valuable in the treatment of hallucinations in dementia with Lewy bodies in particular (McKeith *et al.* 2000, pp.387–92). There would seem to be scope for considering cholinesterase inhibitor use in the confusion of delirium.

Cessation of treatment with cholinesterase inhibitors is also problematic. NICE guidelines (National Institute for Clinical Excellence) advise cessation of treatment below and MMSE (Mini Mental State Examination) of 12/30, yet for the practising clinician, working face to face with the patient and carer, this is less than easy. Formally, withdrawing treatment, observing a rapid decline and recommencing treatment will reintroduce the efficacious impact of the cholinesterase inhibitors but it could be that in the few weeks of that experience a great deal of distress has been caused to patient and carers. The psychological support of the drug treatment is not to be underestimated!

Patterns of NHS old age psychiatry services

The British pattern of old age psychiatry services is that of a service that deals with mental health problems in old age, i.e. organic and functional illness, and not a single specialist dementia service (Fairbairn 2002, pp.423–40). Indeed, there is no drive to change this despite the encouragement of the Alzheimer's Society. This is probably because it was felt that the staff working in such services needed a break from the unremitting and relatively unrewarding care of dementia sufferers. However, today so much more can be offered both medically and socially that one wonders whether the wish for specialist dementia services may well be resurrected.

Organisations within the NHS have an apparent perpetual need to reorganise. The current English pattern of service delivery is large mental health trusts and most old age psychiatry services are within those trusts. However, they probably relate more closely to primary care and local social services than they do to other mental health services. There is therefore an argument that old age psychiatry services might fit best into a primary care trust along with geriatric services. Indeed, combining those services with the older people's element of local social services could create innovative care trusts for older people.

Finally, we might have something to learn from the physicians. Originally, diabetologists were hospital-based physicians, often only with a 'special interest' in diabetes. Now, the management of diabetes is primarily conducted in the community, with specialist teams working closely with primary care and with full-time medical diabetologists. One of the benefits of this is screening, early identification and shared care protocols. Could this be the future for old age psychiatry?

References

Alexopoulos, G.S., Meyers, B.S., Young, R.C., Campbell, S., Silbesweig, D. and Charlson, M. (1997) 'Vascular depression "Hypothesis".' *Archives of General Psychiatry 54*, 915–922.

American Psychiatric Association (1994) *Diagnostic and Statistical Manual*, now DSM IV R. Washington DC: APA.

Anthony, J.C., LeResche, L.A., Von-Korff, M.R., Niaz, U. and Folstien, M.F. (1985) 'Screening for delirium on a general medical ward: the tachistoscope and a global accessibility rating.' *General Hospital Psychiatry 7*, 36–42.

Applegate, W.B., Pressel, S. and Wittes, J. (1994) 'Impact of the treatment of isolated systolic hypertension on behavioural variables. Results from the systolic hypertension in the elderly program.' *Archives of Internal Medicine 154*, 19, 2154–2160.

Arboix, A., Marti-Vilata, J.L. and Garcia, J.H. (1990) 'Clinical study of 222 patients with lacunar infarcts.' *Stroke 21*, 842–847.

Aronson, M.K., Ooi, W.L., Morgernstern, H., Hafner, M.S., Masur, D., Crystal, H., Frishman, W.H., Fisher, D. and Katzman, R. (1990) 'Women, myocardial infarction, and dementia in the very old.' *Neurology 40*, 1102–1106.

Barbro, B.B. (1997) 'Hypertension.' In K.M.A. Welsh, L.R. Caplan, D.J. Reis, B.K. Seisjo and B. Weir (eds) *Primer on Cerebrovascular Diseases*. New York: Academic Press.

Barclay, L.L., Weis, E.M., Mattis, S., Bond, O. and Blass, J.P. (1988) 'Unrecognised cognitive impairment in cardiac rehabilitation patients.' *Journal of American Geriatric Society 36*, 316–325.

Bosch, J., Yusuf, S., Pogue, J., Sleight, P., Lonn, E., Rangoonwala, B., Davies, R., Ostergren, J. and Probstfield, J. (2002) 'Use of ramipril in preventing stroke: double blind randomised trial.' *British Medical Journal 324*, 699–702.

Breteler, M.M.B. (1993) *Cognitive Decline in the Elderly: Epidemiologic Studies on Cognitive Function and Dementia*. Dissertation, Erasmus University.

Brun, A. (1994) 'Pathology and pathophysiology of cerebrovascular dementia: pure subgroups of obstructive and hypoperfusive etiology.' *Dementia 5*, 145–147.

Carmelli, D., Swan, G.E., Reed, T., Mille, B., Wolf, P.A., Jarvik, G.P. and Schellenberg, G.D. (1998) 'Midlife cardiovascular risk factors Apoe E and cognitive decline in elderly male twins.' *Neurology 50*, 6, 1580–1585.

Croxon, S.C.M., Burdon, A.C., Bodington, M. and Botha, J.L. (1991) 'The prevalence of diabetes in elderly people.' *Diabetic Care 8*, 28–31.

Curb, J.D., Rodriguez, B.L., Abbott, R.D., Petrovitch, H., Ross, G.W., Masaki, K.H., Li, C.Y., Curb, J.D., Yano, K., Rodriguez, B.L., Foley, D.J., Blanchette, P.L. and Havlik, R. (1999) 'Longitudinal association of vascular and Alzheimer's dementias, diabetes, and glucose tolerance.' *Neurology 52*, 971–975.

Del Ser, T., Bermejo, F., Portera, A., Arredondo, J.M., Bouros, C. and Constantinidis, J. (1990) 'Vascular dementia: a clinicopathological study.' *Neurology 54*, 1124–1131.

Duppils, G.S. and Wikbald, K. (2001) 'Acute confusional states in patients undergoing hip surgery: a prospective observation study.' *Gerontology 46*, 36–43.

Elias, P.K., Elias, M.F., D'Agostino, R.B., Cupples, L.A., Wilson, P.W., Silbershatz, H. and Wolf, P.A. (1997) 'NIDDM and blood pressure as risk factors for poor cognitive performance: the Framlington study.' *Diabetes Care 20*, 1388–1395.

Elie, M., Cole, M.G., Primeau, F.J. and Bellanvance, F. (1998) 'Delirium risk factors in elderly hospitalised patients.' *Journal of International Medicine 13*, 204–212.

Esiri, M.M., Wilcock, G.K. and Morris, J.H. (1997) 'Neuropathological assessment of the lesions of significance in vascular dementia.' *Journal of Neurology, Neurosurgery, and Psychiatry 63*, 749–753.

Ezekowitz, M.D., James, K.E., Nazarian, S.M., Davenport, J., Broderick, J.P., Gupta, S.R., Thadani, V., Meyer, M.L. and Bridgers, S.L. (1995) 'Silent cerebral infarction in patients with nonrheumatic atrial fibrillation: The Veterans Affairs Stroke Prevention in Nonrheumatic Atrial Fibrillation Investigators.' *Circulation 92*, 2178–2182.

Fairbairn, A. (1997) 'Insight and dementia.' In M. Marshall (ed) *The State of the Art in Dementia*. London: Centre for Policy in Ageing.

Fairbairn, A.F. (2002) 'Principles of service provision in old age psychiatry.' In R. Jacoby and C. Oppenheimer (eds) *Psychiatry in the Elderly*, 3rd edition. Oxford: Oxford University Press.

Farkas, E., De Vos, R.A., Jansen Steur, E.N. and Luiten, P.G. (2000) 'Are Alzheimer's disease, hypertension and cerebrocapillary damage related?' *Neurobiological Ageing 21*, 235–243.

Feinberg, W.M., Seeger, J.F., Carmody, R.K., Anderson, D.C., Hart, R.G. and Pearce, L.A. (1990) 'Epidemiological features of asymptomatic cerebral infarction in patients with nonvalvular atrial fibrillation.' *Archive of International Medicine 150*, 2340–2344.

Fick, D. and Foreman, M. (2000) 'Consequences of not recognising delirium superimposed on dementia in hospitalised elderly individuals.' *Journal of Gerontology Nursing 26*, 30–40.

Fisher, B.W. and Flowerdew, G. (1995) 'A simple model for predicting postoperative delirium in older patients undergoing elective orthopedic surgery.' *Journal of American Geriatric Society 43*, 175–178.

Foreman, M.D. (1989) 'Confusion in the hospitalised elderly: incidence, onset and associated factors.' *Research in Nursing and Health 12*, 21–29.

Forette, F., Seux, M.L., Staessen, J.A., Thijs, L., Birkenhager, W.H., Babarskiene, M.R., Babeanu, S., Bossini, A., Gil Extremera, B., Girerd, X., Laks, T., Lilov, E., Moisseyev, V., Tuomilehto, J., Vanhanen, H., Webster, J., Yodfat, Y. and Fagard, R. (1998) 'Prevention of dementia in randomised double-blind placebo-controlled Systolic Hypertension in Europe (Syst-Eur) trial.' *The Lancet 352*, 1347–1351.

Forette, F., Seux, M.L., Staessen, J.A., Thijs, L., Babarskiene, M.R., Babeanu, S., Bossini, A., Fagard, R., Gil Extremera, B., Laks, T., Kobalava, Z., Sarti, C., Tuomilehto, J., Vanhanen, H., Webster, J., Yodfat, Y. and Birkenhager, W.H. (2002) 'The prevention of dementia with antihypertensive treatment: new evidence from the Systolic Hypertension in Europe (Syst-Eur) study.' *Archives of Internal Medicine 162*, 2046–2052.

Francis, J., Martin, D. and Kapoor, W.N. (1990) 'A prospective study of delirium in hospitalised elderly.' *Journal of the American Medical Association 263*, 1097–1101.

Fujishima, M. and Tsuchihashi, T. (1999) 'Hypertension and dementia.' *Clinical and Experimental Hypertension 21*, 5–6, 927–935.

Gorelick, P.B., Erkinjuntti, T., Hofman, A., Rocca, W.A., Skoog, I. and Winblad, B. (1999) 'Prevention of vascular dementia.' *Alzheimer Disease and Associated Disorders 13*, Suppl 3, SS131–139.

Gregg, E.W., Yaffe, K., Cauley, J.A., Rolka, D.B., Blackwell, T.L., Narayan, K.M. and Cummings, S.R. (2000) 'Is diabetes associated with cognitive impairment and cognitive decline among older women? Study of Osteoporotic Fractures Research Group.' *Archive of International Medicine 160*, 174–180.

Guo, Z., Fratiglioni, L., Viitanen, M., Lannfelt, L., Basun, H., Fastbom, H. and Winblad, B. (2001) 'Apolipoprotein E genotypes and the incidence of Alzheimer's disease among persons aged 75 years and older: variation by use of antihypertensive medication?' *American Journal of Epidemiology 153*, 3, 225–231.

Guo, Z., Viitanen, M., Fratiglioni, L. and Winblad, B. (1996) 'Low blood pressure and dementia in elderly people: the Kungsholmen project.' *British Medical Journal 312*, 805–808.

Hachinski, V.C., Potter, P. and Merskey, H. (1987) 'Leuko-araiosis.' *Archive of Neurology 44*, 21–23.

Hagnell, O., Franck, A., Grasbeck, A., Ohman, R., Ojesjo, L., Otterbeck, L. and Rorsman, B. (1992) 'Vascular dementia in the Lunby study. 1. A prospective epidemiological study of incidence and risk from 1957–1972.' *Neuropsychobiology 26*, 43–49.

Herbert, R., Linsay, J., Verreault, R., Rockwood, K., Hill, G. and Dubois, M.K. (2000) 'Vascular dementia: incidence and risk factors in the Canadian Study of Health and Aging.' *Stroke 31*, 1487–1493.

Hoffman, R.G., Speelman, D.J., Hinnen, D.A., Conley, K.L., Guthrie, R.A. and Knapp, R.K. (1989) 'Changes in cortical functioning with acute hypoglycaemia and hyperglycaemia in type 1 diabetes.' *Diabetes Care 3*, 193–197.

Hogan, D.B., Ebly, E.M. and Rockwood, K. (1997) 'Weight, blood pressure, osmolarity, and glucose levels across various stages of Alzheimer's disease and vascular dementia.' *Dementia and Geriatric Cognitive Disorders 8*, 147–151.

Ince, P.G., McArthur, F.K., Bjertness, E., Torvik, A., Candy, J.M. and Edwardson, J.A. (1995) 'Neuropathological diagnosis of elderly patients in Oslo: Alzheimer's Disease, Lewy bodies disease vascular lesions.' *Dementia 6*, 3, 162–168.

Inouye, S.K. (1999) 'Predisposing and precipitating factors for delirium in hospitalised older patients.' *Dementia and Geriatric Cognitive Disorders 10*, 393–400.

Inouye, S.K. and Charpentier, P.A. (1996) 'Precipitating factors for delirium in hospitalised elderly persons. Predictive model and interrelationship with baseline vulnerability.' *Journal of the American Medical Association 275*, 852–857.

Inouye, S.K., Viscoli, C.M., Horwitz, R.I., Hurtz, L.D. and Tinetti, M.E. (1993) 'A predictive model for delirium in hospitalised elderly medical patients based on admission characteristics.' *Annuals of International Medicine 119*, 474–481.

Jacoby, R. and Oppenheimer, C. (eds) (2002) *Psychiatry in the Elderly*, 3rd edition. Oxford: Oxford University Press.

Jellinger, K., Davidczky, W., Fisher, P., Gabriel, E. (1990) 'Clinicopathological analysis of dementia disorders in the elderly.' *Journal of Neurological Science 95*, 239–258.

Jitapunkel, S., Pillay, I. and Ebrahim, S. (1992) 'Delirium in newly admitted elderly patients: a prospective study.' *Quarterly Journal of Medicine 300*, 307–314.

Johnson, J.C., Gottlieb, G.L., Sullivan, E., Wanich, C., Kinosian, B., Forciea, M.A., Sims, R. and Hoque, C. (1990) 'Using DSM 3 criteria to diagnose delirium elderly general medical patients.' *Journal of Gerontology 45*, MM113–119.

Jorm, A.F. (1990) *The Epidemiology of Alzheimer's Disease and Related Disorders.* London: Chapman and Hall.

Kameyama, M., Fushimi, H. and Udaka, F. (1994) 'Diabetes mellitus and cerebral vascular disease.' *Diabetes Research and Clinical Practice 24*, (suppl), SS205–208.

Kinkel, W.R., Jacobs, L., Polachini, B., Bates, V. and Heffner, R.R. (1985) 'Subcortical arteriosclerotic encephalopathy (Binswanger's disease). Computed tomographic, nuclear magnetic resonance and clinical correlations.' *Neurology 42*, 951–959.

Kivipelto, M., Helkala, E.L., Hallikainen, M., Hanninen, T., Hallikainen, M., Alhainen, K., Livonen, S., Manneraa, A., Tuomilehto, J., Nisinen, A. and Soininen, H. (2000) 'Elevated systolic blood pressure and high cholesterol levels at midlife are risk factors for late life dementia.' *Neurobiological Aging 21*, (suppl 1), S17, abstract.

Kokman, E., Whisnant, J.P., O'Fallon, W.M., Chu, C.P. and Beard, C.M. (1996) 'Dementia after ischaemic stroke: a population based study in Rochester, Minnesota (1960–1984).' *Neurology 46*, 154–159.

Koponen, H.J. and Riekkinen, P.J. (1983) 'A prospective study of delirium in elderly patients admitted to a psychiatric hospital.' *Psychological Medicine 23*, 103–109.

Kuusisto, J., Koivisto, K., Mykkanen, L., Helkala, E.L., Vanhanen, M., Hanninen, T., Kervinen, K., Kesaniemi, Y.A., Riekkinen, P.J. and Laakso, M. (1997) 'Association between features of the insulin resistance syndrome and Alzheimer's disease independently of apolipoprotein ∈ 4 phenotype: cross sectional population based study.' *British Medical Journal 315*, 1045–1049.

Langan, S.J., Deary, I.J., Hepburn, D.A. and Frier, B.M. (1991) 'Cumulative cognitive impairment following recurrent severe hypoglycaemia in adult patients with insulin diabetes mellitus.' *Diabetologia 34*, 337–344.

Launer, L.J., Ross, G.W., Petrovitch, H., Masaki, K., Foley, D., White, L.R. and Havlik, R.J. (2000) 'Midlife blood pressure and dementia: the Honolulu-Asia aging study.' *Neurobiological Aging 21*, 49–55.

Legault, S.E., Joffe, R.T. and Armstrong, P.W. (1992) 'Psychiatric morbidity during early phase of coronary care for myocardial infarction: association with cardiac diagnosis and outcome.' *Canadian Journal of Psychiatry 37*, 316–325.

Leibson, C.L., Rocca, W.A., Hanson, V.A., Cha, A., Kokman, E., O'Brien, P.C. and Palumbo, P.J. (1997) 'Risk of dementia among persons with diabetes mellitus: a population-based cohort study.' *American Journal of Epidemiology 145*, 301–308.

Levkoff, S.E., Evans, D.A., Liptzin, B., Cleary, P.D., Lipsitz, L.A., Wetle, T.T., Reilly, C.H., Pilgrim, D.M. and Rowe, J. (1992) 'Delirium: the occurrence and symptoms among elderly hospitalised patients.' *Archive of International Medicine 152*, 334–340.

Lithell, H., Hansson, L., Skoog, I., Elmfeldt, D., Hofman, A., Olofsson, B., Trenwalder, P. and Zanchetti, A. (2003) 'The Study on Cognition and Prognosis in the Elderly (SCOPE): principal results of a randomised double-blind intervention trial.' *Journal of Hypertension 21*, 875–886.

Lodder, J. and Boiten, J. (1993) 'Incidence, natural history, and risk factors in lacunar infarction.' *Advanced Neurology 62*, 213–227.

Lord Chancellor's Department (1995) *Who Decides? Making Decisions on Behalf of Mentally Incapacitated Adults.* London: HMSO.

Luchsinger, A., Tang, M.X., Stern, Y., Shea, S. and Mayeux, R. (2001) 'Diabetes Mellitus and the risk of Alzheimer's Disease and dementia with stroke in a multiethnic cohort.' *American Journal of Epidemiology 154*, 7, 635–641.

Mankovsky, B.N., Metzger, B.E., Molitch, M.E. and Biller, J. (1992) 'Cerebrovascular disorders in patients with diabetes mellitus.' *Journal of Diabetes Complication 10*, 228–242.

Marcantonio, E.R., Goldman, L., Mangoine, C.M., Ludwig, L.E., Muraca, B., Haslauer, C.M., Donaldson, M.C., Whittmore, A.D., Sugerbaker, D.J. and Poss, R. (1994) 'A clinical prediction rule for delirium after elective non-cardiac surgery.' *Journal of the American Medical Association 271*, 131–139.

Martin, N.J., Stones, M.J., Young, J.E. and Bedard, M. (2000) 'Development of delirium: a prospective cohort study in a community hospital.' *International Psychogeriatrics Society 48*, 618–624.

McKeith, I.G., Grace, J.B., Walker, Z., Byrne, E.J., Wilkinson, D. and Stevens, T. (2000) 'Rivistigmine in the treatment of dementia with Lewy bodies: preliminary findings from an open trial.' *International Journal of Geriatric Psychiatry 15*, 387–392.

Meyer, J.S., Rauch, G., Rauch, R.A. and Haque, A. (2000) 'Risk factors for cerebral hypoperfusion, mild cognitive impairment and dementia.' *Neurobiological Ageing 21*, 161–169.

Murgatroyd, F.D. and Camm, A.J. (1993) 'Atrial arrhythmias.' *Lancet 314*, 1317–1322.

Murray, M.D., Lane, K.A., Gao, S., Evans, R.M., Unverzagt, F.W., Hall, K.S. and Hendrie, H. (2002) 'Preservation of cognitive function with antihypertensive medications: a longitudinal analysis of a community-based sample of African Americans.' *Archives of Internal Medicine 162*, 18, 2090–2096.

Nyenhuis, D.L. and Gorelick, P.B. (1998) 'Vascular dementia: a contemporary review of epidemiology, diagnosis, prevention and treatment.' *Journal of American Geriatric Society 46*, 1473–1478.

O'Brien, J.T., Desmond, P.L., Ames, D., Schweitzer, I., Tuckwell, V. and Tress, B. (1994) 'The differentiation of depression from dementia by temporal lobe magnetic resonance imaging.' *Psychological Medicine 24*, 633–640.

Olichney, J.M., Hansen, L.A., Hofstetter, C.R., Grundman, M., Katzan, R. and Thal, L.J. (1995) 'Cerebral infarct in Alzheimer's disease is associated with severe amyloid angiopathy and hypertension.' *Archive of Neurology 52*, 702–708.

Ott, A., Breteler, M.M., de Bruyne, M.C., van Harskamp, F., Grobbee, D.E. and Hofman, A. (1997) 'Atrial fibrillation and dementia in a population based study. The Rotterdam Study.' *Stroke 28*, 316–321.

Ott, A., Stolk, R.P., van Hardkamp, F., Pols, H.A.P., Hoifman, A., Breteler, M.M.B. (1999) 'Diabetes mellitus and the risk of dementia.' *Neurology 53*, 301–308.

Peila, R., Beatriz, L., Rodriguez, B.L. and Launer, J.L. (2002) 'Type 2 diabetes, Apoe gene and the risk of dementia and related pathologies: the Honolulu-Asia aging study.' *Diabetes 51*, 1256–1262.

Peila, R., White, L.R., Petrovich, H., Maska, K., Ross, G.W., Havlik, R.J. and Launer, L.J. (2001) 'Joint effect of the APOE gene and midlife systolic blood pressure on late-life cognitive impairment: the Honolulu-Asia aging study.' *Stroke 32*, 12, 2882–2889.

Perry, E.K., Perry, R.H., Blessed, G. and Tomlinson, B.E. (1978) 'Changes in brain cholinesterases in senile dementia of Alzheimer's type.' *Neuropathologically Applied Neurobiology 4*, 273–277.

Posner, H.B., Tang, M.X., Luchsinger, J., Lamtigua, R., Stern, Y. and Mayeux, R. (2002) 'The relationship of hypertension in the elderly to AD, vascular dementia, and cognitive function.' *Neurology 58*, 1175–1181.

Pramming, S., Thorsteinsson, B., Theilgaard, A., Pinner, E.M. and Binder, C. (1986) 'Cognitive functioning during hypoglycemia in type 1 diabetes mellitus.' *British Medical Journal 292*, 677–650.

Premkumar, D.R.D., Cohen, D.L., Hedera, P., Friedland, R.P. and Kalaria, R.N. (1996) Apolipoprotein E-∈ 4 alleles in cerebral amyloid angiopathy and cerebrovascular pathology associated with Alzheimer's disease.' *American Journal of Pathology 148*, 6, 2083–2095.

Prince, M.J., Bird, A.S., Blizard, R.A. and Mann, A.H. (1996) 'Is the cognitive function of older patients affected by antihypertensive treatment? Results from 54 months of the Medical Research Council's trial of hypertension in older adults.' *British Medical Journal 312*, 801–805.

The PROGRESS Collaborative Group (2003) 'Effects of blood pressure lowering with perindopril and indapamide therapy on dementia and cognitive decline in patients with cerebrovascular disease.' *Archives of Internal Medicine 163*, 1069–1075.

Rahkonen, T., Luukk-Markkula, R., Paanila, S., Sivenius, J. and Sulkava, T. (2000) 'Delirium episode as assign of undetected dementia among community dwelling elderly subjects: a 2 year follow up study.' *Journal of Neurology, Neurosurgery and Psychiatry 69*, 519–521.

Reich, P., Regestein, Q.R., Murawski, B.J., DeSilva, R.A. and Lown, B. (1983) 'Unrecognised organic mental disorders in survivors of cardiac arrest.' *American Journal of Psychiatry 140*, 119–1197.

Rockwood, K. (1994) 'The occurrence and duration of symptoms in elderly patients with delirium.' *Journal of Gerontology Medicine Science 42*, 252–256.

Rockwood, K., Cosway, S., Carver, D., Jarret, P., Stadnyk, K. and Fisk, J. (1999) 'The risk of dementia and death after delirium.' *Age and Aging 28*, 551–556.

Rolfson, D.B., McElhaney, J.E., Rockwood, K., Finnegan, B.A., Entwistle, L.M., Wong, J.F. and Almazor, M.E. (1999) 'Incidence and risk factors for delirium and other adverse outcomes in older adults after coronary artery bypass graft surgery.' *Canadian Journal of Cardiology 15*, 771–776.

Roman, G.C., Tatemichi, T., Erkinjuntti, T., Cummings, J.L., Masden, J.C. and Garcia, J.H. (1993) 'Vascular dementia: diagnostic criteria for research studies. Report of the NINCDS AIRENS international workshop.' *Neurology 43*, 250–260.

Ryan, C.M., Williams, T.M., Finegold, D.N. and Orchard, T.J. (1993) 'Cognitive dysfunction in adults with type 1 (insulin dependent) diabetes mellitus of long duration: effects of recurrent hypoglycaemia and other complications.' *Diabetologia 36*, 329–344.

Skoog, I., Lernfelt, B., Landahl, S., Palmertz, B., Andreasson, L.A., Nilsson, L., Persson, G., Oden, A. and Svanborg, A. (1996) '15 year longitudinal study of blood pressure in dementia.' *Lancet 347*, 1141–1145.

Slater, E. and Roth, M. (1969) *Clinical Psychiatry*, 3rd edition. London: Baillière Tindall and Cassell.

Snowden, D.A., Greiner, L.H., Mortimer, J.A., Riley, K.P., Greiner, P.A. and Markesbery, W.R. (1997) 'Brain infarction and the clinical expression of Alzheimer's disease: the nun study.' *Journal of the American Medical Association 277*, 813–817.

Soneira, C.F. and Scott, T.M. (1998) 'Severe cardiovascular disease and Alzheimer's disease: senile plaque formation in cortical areas.' *Clinical Anatomy 9*, 2, 118–127.

Sparks, D.L., Hunsaker, J.C., Scheff, S.W., Kryscio, R.J., Sparks, D.L., Hunsaker, J.C., Scheff, S.W., Kryscio, R.J., Henson, J.L. and Markesbery, W.R. (1990) 'Cortical senile plaques in coronary artery disease, aging and Alzheimer's disease.' *Neurobiology of Aging 11*, 6, 601–607.

Stegmayr, B. and Asplund, K. (1995) 'Diabetes a risk factor for stroke: a population perspective.' *Diabetologia 38*, 1061–1068.

Stewart, R.B., Moore, M.T., May, F.E., Marks, R.G. and Hale, W.E. (1991) 'Correlates of cognitive dysfunction in an ambulatory elderly population.' *Gerontology 37*, 272–280.

Strachan, M.W.J., Deary, I.J., Ewing, F.M.E. and Frier, B.M. (1997) 'Is type II diabetes associated with an increased risk of cognitive dysfunction?' *Diabetes Care 20*, 438–445.

Tatemichi, T.K., Paik, M., Bagiella, E., Desmond, D.W., Stern, Y., Sano, M., Hauser, W.A. and Mayeux, R. (1994) 'Risk of dementia after stroke in a hospitalised cohort: results of a longitudinal study.' *Neurology 44*, 1885–1891.

Tavornen-Schroder, S., Roytta, M., Raiha, I., Kurki, T., Rajala, T. Sourander, L. (1996) 'Clinical features of leuko-araiosis.' *Journal of Neurology, Neurosurgery and Psychiatry 60*, 431–436.

Victoroff, J., Mack, W.J., Lyness, S.A. and Chui, H.C. (1995) 'Multicentre clinicopathological correlations in dementia.' *American Journal of Psychiatry 152*, 10, 1476–1484.

Werner, P., Cohen-Mansfield, E.B., Braun, J. and Marx, M.S. (1989) 'Physical restraints and agitation in nursing home residents.' *Journal of American Geriatric Society 37*, 1122–1126.

Williams, M.A., Campbell, E.B., Raynor, W.J., Musholt, M.A., Mlynarczyk, S.M. and Crane, L.F. (1985) 'Predictors of acute confusional states in hospitalised elderly patients.' *Research in Nursing and Health 8*, 31–40.

Williams-Russo, P., Urquhart, B.L., Sharrock, N.E. and Chisholm, M.E. (1992) 'Post operative delirium: predictors and prognosis in elderly orthopaedic patients.' *Journal of American Geriatrics Society 40*, 759–767.

Ylikoski, A., Erkinjuntti, T., Raininko, R., Sarna, R., Sulkava, R. and Tilvis, R. (1995) 'White matter hyperintensities on MRI in the neurologically non-diseased elderly: analysis of cohorts of consecutive subjects aged 55 to 85 years living at home.' *Stroke 26*, 1171–1177.

Yoshitake, T., Kiyohara, Y., Kato, I., Ohmura, T., Iwamoto, H., Nakayama, K., Ohmori, S., Nomiyama, K., Kawano, H. and Ueda, K. (1995) 'Incidence and risk factors of vascular dementia and Alzheimer's disease in a defined elderly Japanese population: the Hisayama study.' *Neurology 45*, 1161–1168.

Zuccala, G., Cattel, C., Manes-Gravina, E., Di Nero, M.G., Cocchi, A. and Bernabei, R. (1997) 'Left ventricular dysfunction: a clue to cognitive heart impairment in older patients with heart failure.' *Journal of Neurology, Neurosurgery and Psychiatry 63*, 509–512.

CHAPTER 14

Social Science Theory on Dementia Research: Normal Ageing, Cultural Representation and Social Exclusion

John Bond, Lynne Corner and Ruth Graham

Age stratification and institutionalised ageism are widespread across the world. Human life-spans are increasing steadily world-wide (United Nations 2000), mainly as a result of improvements in living conditions, sanitation and healthcare (Coleman and Bond 1993). With the success of this demographic revolution has been the corresponding increase in the number of older people with Alzheimer's disease or other types of dementia (Alzheimer's Disease International 2000). Dementia is a truly global phenomenon within the context of cultural, economic and social globalisation.

This chapter investigates the marginalisation of people with dementia from critical gerontological and sociological perspectives with a view to increasing our understanding. Along the way we will define our concepts and place them within a broader sociological framework (see also Bond 2001). The argument to be presented can be summarised as follows. Age is just one way in which human societies are stratified (Riley, Johnson and Finer 1972). In most cultures older people are marginalised and socially excluded on the basis of age. But many older people are oppressed not just by their age but also because of their gender, ethnic and class background (Arber and Ginn 1991b; Hulko 2002). People with dementia are further excluded because they lack cognitive citizenship (Graham 2004). Cultural representations of people with dementia, like those of older people in general, are essentially negative (Manthorpe 2000). They, at the same time, reflect the negative stereotypes of old age and dementia and reinforce institutionalised ageism (Bytheway and Johnson 1991) and the exclusion of people with dementia. Despite the adoption of principles of personhood (Kitwood 1997), people with dementia continue to be stigmatised (Goffman 1968) and be part of oppressive caring relationships in which their perspectives are subservient to those of others around them (Harris 2002a). Physical and mental decline in later life is widely perceived as normal by older people, their families and many health professionals. But contemporary thinking in biomedical science is that many of the vicissitudes of old age are pathological (Kirkwood 1999). The biomedical approach and the subsequent medicalisation of dementia (Bond 1992a; Bond *et al.* 2002) further excludes older people with dementia who become increasingly commodified as biomedical scientists seek their 'Nobel prizes' and biotechnology and pharmaceutical industries market their products (Estes *et al.* 2001). Returning true personhood, including autonomy and control, to older people with dementia is a way to increase social inclusion.

The social position of older people in society

Seeking to understand social structures has been a core activity of sociology since its emergence as a distinct social science some time during the 19th century. Social stratification theory, however, focused for many years almost exclusively on class relations (Giddens 1973), to the exclusion of other dimensions of inequality. Even within a political economy perspective early texts excluded the importance of gender, ethnicity and disability (Jenkins 1991; Phillipson 1982; Townsend 1981; Walker 1980, 1981). In recent years the impact of feminism and the social science response to racism has been reflected in social stratification theory (Abbott and Wallace 1990; Giddens and Birdsall 2001) and the political economy of old age (Arber and Ginn 1991a; Estes *et al.* 2001; Fennell, Phillipson and Evers 1988; Phillipson 1998).

The hegemony of class in social stratification theory reflects the role of paid work as a central tenet of 19th-century patriarchal capitalist societies. It also helps explain the exclusion of gender in stratification theory. In understanding the position of older people in modern society, paid work remains an important organising principle and explanation of income inequality. The position of an older person reflects their position as a younger member of society. Their class position and the development of human and social capital will have been determined by their position in the labour market throughout their working lives. Education and social background, gender and ethnic status, and mental or physical impairment will have been of influence in determining their role in the labour market. The economic, political and social dominance of 'white', middle-class men within post-colonial capitalist society throughout recent history means that the majority of older people are oppressed by virtue of their female gender, minority ethnic status and social class position. Physical and mental decline further increases the experience of 'intersectionality' among older people or people with dementia (Hulko 2002). An older person's position or locale in the social structure therefore generally militates against social inclusion and denies them full practical social rights as citizens.

But in understanding social exclusion we need to go beyond issues of structure and social categories. We need to reflect on our understanding of human or individual agency. Agency embodies not only ideas from social action theory (Gerth and Mills 1948, p.28) and explanations of objective human action in terms of intention and rationality (Mead 1934). Agency is also about individual action, which is passionate and intuitive and distinctly subjective (Lash and Urry 1986). In post modernity we increasingly see ourselves as individuals within a consumer society, which emphasises 'lifestyle' rather than the traditional structural contexts of class, gender and ethnicity. Postmodernist writers argue that our personal identities are increasingly 'expressed, revised and represented through consumption' (Gilleard and Higgs 2000). If this is the case social exclusion is simply exclusion from a desired lifestyle and consumption pattern while practical citizenship focuses on the social rights of individuals to choose lifestyles of their choice.

Thus in contemporary debates about social exclusion a key issue has been how to create opportunities for agency that allow individuality and subjectivity in social action, for people defined as socially vulnerable such as older people and particularly people with cognitive impairments. In our 'hypercognitive culture' (Post 1995) older people with dementia are generally not expected to fulfil the expectations of rationality, intention or indeed to maintain a sense of identity or personhood. This perspective has been widely challenged by people with dementia, practitioners and 'dementia' researchers in the wake of the late Tom Kitwood's persuasive and honourable crusade to re-establish personhood in dementia (Kitwood 1997).

Graham (2004) has observed that people with dementia are socially excluded because their citizenship rights necessarily depend on their abilities to act with agency and develop a continuing sense of self and personal identity. It is this lack of *cognitive citizenship* among people with dementia, rather than the presence of opportunities or resources, that increases their social exclusion and marginalisation. The challenge therefore remains how to increase social inclusion and preserve the practical social rights of people with cognitive impairment or dementia. Given the prevailing image in post modernity of the social incompetence of people with dementia one approach is to work on the cultural representation of dementia.

Cultural representation of dementia

Images of older people and of people with dementia are represented through oral and written language as well as other media such as photographs and film. Of course, as Blaikie and Hepworth (1997) assert, images are only a symbolic representation of reality, representative of a particular symbolic order and defined within a specific culture or society. For example, within contemporary capitalist consumer society images of the human body such as wrinkles, grey hair and baldness are central to our cultural representation of ageing. They are treated as a sign of corporeal and moral decay. But the wrinkle on the face of a Chinese grandmother is greeted with joy because it is a sign of high status (Featherstone and Hepworth 1993, p.306).

There does exist in the public's perception, however, a view that ageing is a bodily affair and that the development of wrinkles, grey hair and balding is evidence of human ageing. This common-sense knowledge of our bodies, biomedical focus on the biological body and the development of a consumer culture and commercial interest in keeping the body fit, slim, young and 'beautiful' highlights the symbolic significance of our bodily state and increases the commodification of ageing individuals' fears and desires (Gilleard and Higgs 2000; Sawchuk 1995). The physical appearance of the ageing body has never been venerated. As in earlier times, wealth and power remain the main source of reverence (Laslett 1977). In their influential overview of traditional and modern images of ageing, Featherstone and Hepworth (1993) make the distinction between the 'good old', 'bad old' and those who are 'simply past it' (Box 14.1). Their category 'simply past it' includes people with dementia.

The negative stereotypes of old age reflected in 'simply past it' build on the contrast between the ideal of the fit body of youth and the ageing body. Overlaying the beauty of the body is that of cognitive ability in our 'hypercognitive' world. Such symbolic polarities, like the use of black and white in everyday language, are not fixed and will change with changes in

---

Box 14.1 Traditional images of later life

Good old – wise, passive, moral and affable

Bad old – reject above stereotypes

Simply past it – frail, 'senile', geriatric

---

context and over time. But stereotypes of older people go beyond the simple images of the ageing body and, for older people with dementia, beyond the incompetence of the ageing mind. They incorporate moral interpretations of 'normal ageing' reflected in physical and cognitive decline to describe behavioural and attitudinal aspects. Butler (1987) in his formulation of ageism suggests that older people are perceived as senile, rigid in thought and manner, and old-fashioned in morality and skills. Most of these stereotypes are negative.

The lived experience of dementia

An important aspect of the cultural representation of dementia and the inherent negative stereotyping of older people and older people with dementia is the stigmatising effect on everyday interactions and the quality of life they experience. There have been a number of accounts of this 'lived experience of dementia' (Lyman 1998) in personal accounts (Friedell 2002; Sterin 2002), biographies (Bayley 1998; McGown 1993) and novels (Bernlef 1984; Forster 1989), as well as in primary research (Gubrium 1987; Harris 2002a, 2002b; Sabat 2001). These studies highlight the often oppressive nature of caring relationships in which the perspectives of people with dementia are subservient to those of others around them, as can be illustrated by selected material from the following case study which has been discussed elsewhere (Bond *et al.* 2002) to illustrate ideas about lack of insight in dementia and to reflect on lay concepts of risk. We can also use the case study to illustrate other aspects of social theory: labelling theory and the sociology of deviance, stigma and the medicalisation of dementia. Of course this case study is only illustrative. Alone it is not explanatory.

Dennis and Margaret

At the time of the case study Dennis and Margaret (pseudonyms) had been married for 35 years. They lived in a modern terraced house, which had been adapted to suit Margaret's needs. She had severe arthritis and oedema in her legs, and while she could walk around the house with the aid of two sticks, she found it difficult to get up from a chair alone. Margaret remained independent, but only because she had a stair lift and used an electric wheelchair to get about outside of the home.

Dennis was an athlete and keen gardener. His physical build was lean and slight and it was not hard on meeting him to imagine him pounding the pavements pursuing his passion for long-distance running. For over 35 years he had been an active member of a local running club, training with fellow members for marathons, completing daily training runs and exercising in the gym. Through the running club, he had competed throughout his long career, completing over 25 half marathons and, the crowning of his achievements, completing a local marathon in three hours, ten minutes. The running club also constituted a major part of his social life. He and fellow members met once a week in a local pub and he had developed many close friendships with other club members. Running was clearly important to his quality of life and to his sense of identity. Keeping physically fit was also hugely important to him. He eloquently described the sense of freedom he had always felt when running, how he found running relaxing and how he cleared his mind, running on 'auto-pilot'. The sense of achievement he felt when completing a run was 'fantastic'.

> Your body feels good all the time, that's what it feels like, it drives you on because you are wanting to do that all the time and get faster. (Interview 2, page 19, line 18)

Dennis had been experiencing memory problems for six years when he was diagnosed with probable Alzheimer's. The impact of the stigma of the disease on Dennis' life was immediate. Shortly after diagnosis Dennis withdrew from running. Friends from the local club no longer contacted him to join them. This had been particularly hurtful to Dennis and he had felt unable to contact his friends, and his closest friend in particular, for an explanation as to why the contact had ceased. Margaret explained:

> ...a friend of his, a very good friend actually, they've been running for years together, came out and saw him last year and said 'Right, Dennis, I'm still running...I'll come and pick you up and I'll take you and I'll bring you back, give us a ring if you want to go.' So, I says 'Do you want to go?' 'Yes.' So I rang and told him he wanted to go and he never rang back and that really, really upset him. I don't think he ever got over that yet. (Interview 1, page 9, line 1)

Margaret described the effect that this incident had had on Dennis:

> I think he's frightened of getting let down again, you know…he's frightened
> to trust again. (Interview 1, page 9, line 27)

Margaret felt Dennis could no longer go out running by himself, focusing on
the risks involved and the potential consequences. She expressed her fear of
him being hurt, getting lost and being unable to find his way home. Dennis
said that he wished he could still run, and felt that he still could. Physically he
remained fit and lean; still the body of an athlete. But others had placed
restrictions on his choices and excluded him from his lifetime favourite
pastime. He had been denied practical citizenship because of his cognitive
abilities.

No known attempt was made to facilitate his enjoyment of running. For
example, there was an enclosed park nearby. Margaret deemed this to be an
'unacceptable risk'. Professionals legitimised the caregiver's feelings, and no
attempts were made to take on board just how important running was to Dennis' self-concept. The increasing emphasis on his cognitive deficits had a huge
effect on his quality of life, and a catastrophic effect on how he perceived
himself.

Dennis and Margaret were both keen gardeners. Dennis had always
enjoyed pottering in the garden, but the pleasure from what was once a particularly enjoyable activity had been diminished because he felt 'hemmed in' in
the garden. He continued to have lots of energy and was 'always on the go'.
The energy that he once diverted into running had nowhere to be channelled,
leaving him feeling frustrated and empty.

> He's like a bear with a sore head if he can't get outside. Paces the floor and
> drives me mad because…if he's in the house he's on top of me all the time.
> (Interview 3, page 10, line 51)

Dennis expressed how he enjoyed watching seeds grow. He enjoyed watching
them 'come on' over the winter in the large greenhouse in the back garden:

> I think it's the flowers, watching them grow. (Interview 3, page 15, line 31)

> Why you can, how can I put it, it's er, watching the plants and your er see
> plants they want mixing, want doing. (Interview 3, page 31, line 11)

> I like watching them come on, ye nah, from nowt up to, well, plants, yer nah.
> (Interview 4, page 3, line 17)

During the first visit to the couple, Dennis was a touchingly enthusiastic host,
eagerly showing off his seeds planted in neat rows of trays on shelves around

the greenhouse. His wife remarked on that same day that the greenhouse was going to be taken down as she was concerned that Dennis would walk through the glass and she was frightened that he would hurt himself:

> That's [greenhouse] going. End of next week. There's someone from the council coming to take it away. I just sit waiting for the crash…of him losing his balance and falling through and… (Interview 2, page 17, line 20)

She said that she knew that Dennis did not want the greenhouse to go, but felt that with the risks involved this was inevitable. Margaret also felt that Dennis did not have insight into the risks that she perceived:

> Oh no, no, he doesn't want it to go, no. But he can't see you see, he doesn't understand. (Interview 2, page 17, line 34)

When Dennis and Margaret were next visited, two weeks later, the greenhouse had gone. Margaret also felt that Dennis over-watered all the plants in the garden and so a few months ago had arranged for all the flowerbeds to be gravelled. A range of containers replaced them. She perceived that these would be easier to manage. Dennis thought it looked grey and bland, although he remained optimistic about the new challenge of planting the containers to bring colour into the garden:

> Aye it's given me summat to think on, aye, get some colour in them, get some colour in. (Interview 3, page 2, line 6)

Despite the fact that Margaret was very concerned about the risks to Dennis when he was out and about, equally Dennis was concerned about Margaret. They were regular visitors to the local garden centre and Dennis described what he did not like about the journey there. His concerns related to the problems he perceived with Margaret's electric wheelchair running out of power, because of the number of hills on the journey:

> I'm always frightened when we're getting it [wheelchair] out in the entrance, there er, er, we gan up to the edge because there's not much around there once it's up. (Interview 3, page 33, line 34)

Stigma and dementia

We have already seen the stigmatising effect that a diagnosis of dementia had on Dennis with the exclusion by his friends from running. Goffman (1968) refers to stigma as a relationship of devaluation in which one individual is disqualified from full social acceptance. Stigma is a social attribute that is discrediting for an individual or group. It seems likely that people with dementia would be stigmatised because of the 'out of the ordinary' (Dingwall 1976) or problematic behaviours of those with dementia. The bizarre behaviours characteristic of people with the disease clearly challenge social norms regarding appropriate conduct and it is likely that it was the expectation of such behaviour that kept Dennis' friends away.

Our negative stereotypes of people with dementia reflect each of three types of stigma first delineated by Goffman (1968). Images of physical and cognitive impairments – wrinkles, baldness, stooping, limping, failing memory and bizarre behaviour – are stigmatised characteristics of individuals. 'Blemishes of individual character' such as being rigid in thought and old-fashioned are inferred. Even the 'tribal' behaviour of different generations produces stigmatised effects. A ubiquitous feature of the stigmatising of individuals is the development of a negative discourse. We use specific words in everyday life such as 'wrinkly', 'crumbly', 'grouchy', 'gaga', 'senile' and 'biddy' as metaphors, without giving thought to their original meaning. And we tend to impute a wide range of imperfections on the basis of the original meaning of the word – a process which reinforces negative stereotypes. Noticeably such terms are not restricted to the use by younger people; older people also hold strong stereotypes of others of the same age or generation (Giles and Coupland 1991). Attempts to introduce 'political correctness' in our everyday language about people with dementia will probably fail until our underlying images and stereotypes of people with dementia change and we overcome institutionalised ageism.

There is an absence of research-based evidence of the presence of stigma in dementia (Macrae 1999) but this may reflect the nature of the disease in which people with dementia may not be aware of others' negative response to their behaviour. However, biographical accounts, written by people who were in the early stages of dementia, indicate that some individuals experienced embarrassment and shame (McGown 1993).

Stigma remains a major barrier to increased participation, both for the person with dementia and for their informal caregiver. Therefore in practice we need to identify ways of neutralising the effects of stigma if we wish to achieve the aim of greater social participation for this marginalised group in our society. It will be at the societal level where most change must occur. The publicity generated by advocates of people with dementia and the coming out of celebrities with dementia will have greatest impact on making dementia a less discreditable condition.

Labelling theory

The case study of Dennis and Margaret provides an excellent illustration of labelling theory and the operation of primary and secondary deviance (Lemert 1964). Labelling is a social process by which individuals or groups classify the social behaviour of other individuals. Psychiatric diagnoses are particularly good examples of the process since they normally have behavioural as well as organic or physical components and those supplying the label have been legitimised by society to do so. Thus dementia is a classic example of primary deviance. In our hypercognitive society memory loss is increasingly seen as a deviant attribute. Although contested within the scientific community (Huppert, Brayne and O'Connor 1994), brain ageing and memory impairment is defined as pathological and not a normal ageing process. The deviant behaviour is understood to have an underlying physical pathology which can only be identified by those with the authority to make clinical diagnoses. A diagnosis of dementia has significance within post modernity because of the power of the medical profession to make such diagnoses. A lay diagnosis of dementia may not be so enduring. In the case of Dennis and Margaret memory impairment was recognised by them both and it is likely that many of Dennis' fellow runners observed the symptoms of what was eventually diagnosed as Alzheimer's disease. The accounts of the couple, however, suggest that this was treated as relatively normal for a man of Dennis' age.

For Dennis the most important impact of receiving the diagnosis of Alzheimer's disease was the effect the label had on others around him. The process of secondary deviance appeared to be rapid. The formal diagnosis allowed Margaret to take a fuller control over Dennis' life as illustrated by the removal of the greenhouse and changes to the garden. His friends deserted him and he became even more dependent on Margaret. Although not presented in this account it is not unusual for people given the label of demented or senile to take on some of the behaviours associated with the condition (Bond 2001).

Normal ageing and the biomedicalisation of dementia

Although contested (Kay and Roth 2002), recent epidemiological data (Neuropathology Group of the Medical Research Council Cognitive Function and Ageing Study 2001) suggest that the boundary between normal ageing and cognitive impairment is not as clear cut as often claimed by biomedical scientists demarcating the boundaries between normal and pathological brain ageing and between cultural beliefs and scientific facts. The 'boundary work' (Gieryn 1983, 1995) of biomedical scientists focuses on Popperian epistemological practices of theory falsification (Popper 1961). For Popper scientific method is not about confirmation and verification of theory in which the scientist seeks evidence to corroborate a generalisation but rather about falsification in which the scientist seeks evidence to refute it. He arrived at this epistemological position through his analysis of Freudian psychoanalysis and Marxism, arguing that, once you arrive at a theoretical position using verification as the guiding principle, confirming instances of a particular theory appear everywhere. In other words there is a danger that verification leads to selective identification and interpretation of available empirical evidence.

The challenge for the biomedical scientist is to provide reproducible evidence to falsify scientific predictions. Constructionists contested the infallibility of the Popperian philosophy of science by challenging the reproducibility of falsifying empirical evidence. Falsifiability is a logical condition that requires the practical accomplishment of observation and experiment. Constructionists did not challenge these premises but argued that practical everyday science is surrounded by interpretative ambiguities that get resolved through complex social and often political negotiations. Thus an essential question for scientists and constructionists alike is: when is an empirical scientific statement replicated, reproduced or corroborated (Collins 1985)? The answer to this question becomes one on which scientists and others continue to negotiate.

In clinical practice diagnosis remains a professional judgement based on scientific knowledge and professional beliefs. Diagnosis of psychiatric conditions appears a very uncertain science. Although there are agreed clinical algorithms for the identification of cognitive impairment and diagnosis of dementia based on professional consensus, in practice reproducibility is inconsistent. The reliability of psychiatric diagnosis has been widely contested and in the absence of falsifiable biological markers will remain so. Traditional clinical assessments of cognition are far from reliable between observers and over time at the individual level. Many of the measures currently used fail to reach consensus standards of psychometric reliability and validity at the population level. Thus theories about normal cognitive ageing have not been robustly falsified. There is, however, increasing professional consensus that alternative models of cognitive ageing based on pathological brain ageing provide convincing explanations of the human behaviours associated with a diagnosis of dementia. But many of these models are built on the verification principle. Like theories of normal cognitive ageing in human subjects principles of falsification have not been robustly applied.

Biomedical science has often been challenged for the medicalisation of everyday life through the subordination of lay and cultural beliefs to professional and expert scientific power. The questions of importance here are not about whether cognitive impairment is a normal part of human ageing. Rather it is about how medicalisation of cognitive impairment leads to social exclusion and the marginalisation of dementia. And how does the pathologisation and problematisation of dementia reinforce social exclusion and deny cognitive citizenship? Although well documented elsewhere, reviewing the process of medicalisation in dementia and the role of scientists in the development of scientific knowledge may contribute to providing an answer to these questions.

Medicalisation of dementia

Medicalisation is the process of defining behaviour as a medical problem and mandating the medical profession to establish biological causes and cures and provide treatments for it. The medicalisation of disease in general (Conrad 1975; Estes and Binney 1989; Freidson 1975) and cognitive impairment and dementia (Bond 1992a, 1992b, 2001; Bond et al. 2002; Lyman 1989) has been well documented. In brief there are four essential aspects: expert control (Freidson 1975), social control (Zola 1972), individualisation of behaviour and de-politicisation of behaviour. Doctors are the experts and they have a monopoly over medical knowledge and control diagnosis and treatment. It is the psychiatrist who has the power to legitimise the social status of normal or pathological. Individualisation of behaviour seeks explanations and solutions of dementia in the individual rather than the broader social context leading to the 'blaming' of the individual (Oliver 1996). De-politicisation of behaviour ignores the meaning of dementia to the individual that goes beyond loss of cognitive function. Thus the process of medicalisation denies that the person with dementia can experience personhood and a sense of self (Davis 2003) and reinforces social exclusion.

The role of science

Scientists create boundaries between scientific and non-scientific activities in order to pursue a number of personal professional goals (Gieryn 1983). These include the establishment and maintenance of a funded and intellectually interesting scientific career; the control of expert power over the intellectual content of science and scientific method; control of scientific resources and denial of these resources to non-scientists or 'pseudoscientists'; and the protection of the autonomy of scientists and scientific activity from political interference. The nature of science and its involvement with society is forever changing and scientific boundaries are drawn and redrawn within the changing historical, economic, political and social context. Within this context the primary goal of biomedical science is not to seek cures and treatments for the population of ill people but to achieve personal fulfilment for individual scientists within their professional lives. Biomedical science can be seen as an end in itself.

In post modernity the role of biomedical science is on the one hand predominant in the social lives of citizens through the process of medicalisation, but on the other hand is increasingly being subsumed by the hegemony of the medical-industrial complex. The medical-industrial complex refers to the multi-billion pound healthcare industry made up of health professionals, hospitals, nursing homes, community health services, insurance companies, drug, device and equipment manufacturers, and the construction and financial service industries. The nature of contemporary healthcare industry suggests that its main function is the pursuit of profit rather than the delivery of services (Ehrenreich and Ehrenreich 1970). The increasingly globalised medical-industrial complex is increasingly challenging the autonomy and authority of health professionals concerning health and illness and is subsuming the activities of science in the pursuit of profit. Thus, like the caring professions, medical scientists have lost scientific autonomy and control over scientific knowledge.

Recent advances in scientific knowledge about the causes and treatment of dementia have increased the commodification of dementia and reinforced the social exclusion and marginalisation of people with dementia. 'Commodification is the process of taking a good or service that has been produced and used, but not bought or sold, and turning it into an item that is exchanged for money' (Estes *et al.* 2001, p.49). For example the bathing of people with dementia by family carers within their own homes does not involve a commodity relationship, but the purchasing of this service from a private provider commodifies the task. In the case of dementia commodification has been characterised by the increase in the use of resources to seek treatments for dementia without real corresponding increases in the resources given to people with dementia and their supporting families.

Barriers to social inclusion

Critical gerontology provides a range of perspectives on the process of ageing in contemporary European societies and provides a sociological understanding of the marginalisation of people with dementia. In this chapter we have reviewed a number of barriers to increasing the social inclusion of older people with dementia. At the interpersonal level, the hegemony of institutionalised ageism and the negative cultural presentation of older people in society remains a major barrier and reinforces negative attitudes, the stigmatisation of people with dementia and the experience of primary and secondary deviance. The social position and the experience of inter-sectionality of older people with dementia militates against acting with agency and denies them cognitive citizenship. The dominant ageist, sexist, racist and disablist cultural values are a barrier to achieving personhood. At a societal level the power of medical science to control our understanding of normal and pathological further marginalises the person with dementia. But reinforcing all these trends is the hegemony of the globalised medical-industrial complex that continues to subserve all human needs in the pursuit of the capitalist goals of profit.

Understanding the marginalisation of people with dementia has been the purpose of this chapter rather than practical suggestions for achieving cognitive citizenship and personhood. In practical terms, however, perhaps the only mechanism available to improving the status of people with dementia will be through the evangelical work of writers such as Kitwood and Post and through the international efforts of members of social movements like the International Alzheimer's Association. These efforts have made a difference, but there is still a long way to go before older people with dementia achieve true citizenship in our contemporary world.

References

Abbott, P. and Wallace, C. (1990) *An Introduction to Sociology: Feminist Perspectives.* London: Routledge.

Alzheimer's Disease International (2000) *Annual Report 1999–2000.* London: Alzheimer's Disease International.

Arber, S. and Ginn, J. (1991a) *Gender and Later Life: A Sociological Analysis of Resources and Constraints.* London: Sage Publications.

Arber, S. and Ginn, J. (1991b) 'The invisibility of age: gender and class in later life.' *Sociological Review 39,* 260–291.

Bayley, J. (1998) *Iris: A Memoir of Iris Murdoch.* London: Duckworth.

Bernlef, J. (1984) *Out of Mind.* London: Faber and Faber.

Blaikie, A. and Hepworth, M. (1997) 'Representations of old age in painting and photography.' In A. Jamieson, S. Harper and C. Victor (eds) *Critical Approaches to Ageing and Later Life.* Buckingham: Open University Press.

Bond, J. (1992a) 'The medicalisation of dementia.' *Journal of Aging Studies 6,* 397–403.

Bond, J. (1992b) 'The politics of care-giving: the professionalisation of informal support.' *Ageing and Society 12,* 5–21.

Bond, J. (2001) 'Sociological perspectives.' In C. Cantley (ed) *A Handbook of Dementia Care.* Buckingham: Open University Press.

Bond, J., Corner, L., Lilley, A. and Ellwood, C. (2002) 'Medicalisation of insight and caregivers' response to risk in dementia.' *Dementia 1,* 3, 313–328.

Butler, R.N. (1987) 'Ageism.' In *The Encyclopaedia of Aging.* New York: Springer.

Bytheway, B. and Johnson, J. (1991) 'On defining ageism.' *Critical Social Policy 27,* 27–39.

Coleman, P. and Bond, J. (1993) 'Ageing in the twentieth century.' In J. Bond, P. Coleman and S. Peace (eds) *Ageing in Society: An Introduction to Social Gerontology,* 2nd edition. London: Sage.

Collins, H.M. (1985) *Changing Order: Replication and Induction in Scientific Practice.* London: Sage.

Conrad, P. (1975) 'The discovery of Hyperkinesis: notes on the medicalisation of deviant behaviour.' *Social Problems 23,* 1, 12–21.

Davis, D.H.J. (2004) 'Dementia: sociological and philosophical constructions.' *Social Science and Medicine 58,* 369–378.

Dingwall, R. (1976) *Aspects of Illness.* London: Martin Robertson.

Ehrenreich, J. and Ehrenreich, B. (1970) *The American Health Empire: Power, Profits and Politics.* New York: Random House.

Estes, C.L. and Binney, E. (1989) 'The biomedicalisation of aging: dangers and dilemmas.' *Gerontologist 29,* 5, 587–596.

Estes, C.L., Alford, R.R., Binney, E.A., Bradsher, J.E., Close, L., Collins, C.A., Egan, A.H., Harrington, C., Linkins, K.W., Lynch, M., Mahakian, J.L., Pellow, D.N., Wallace, S.P. and Weitz, T.A. (2001) *Social Policy and Aging: A Critical Perspective.* Thousand Oaks: Sage.

Featherstone, M. and Hepworth, M. (1993) 'Images of ageing.' In J. Bond, P. Coleman and S. Peace (eds) *Ageing in Society: An Introduction to Social Gerontology,* 2nd edition. London: Sage.

Fennell, G., Phillipson, C. and Evers, H. (1988) *The Sociology of Old Age.* Milton Keynes: Open University Press.

Forster, M. (1989) *Have the Men Had Enough?* London: Penguin Books.

Freidson, E. (1975) *Profession of Medicine: A Study of the Sociology of Applied Knowledge.* New York: Dodd, Mead and Co.

Friedell, M. (2002) 'Awareness: a personal memoir on the declining quality of life in Alzheimer's.' *Dementia 1,* 3, 359–366.

Gerth, H.H. and Mills, C.W. (1948) *From Max Weber: Essays in Sociology.* London: Routledge and Kegan Paul.

Giddens, A. (1973) *The Class Structure of the Advanced Societies.* London: Hutchinson.

Giddens, A. and Birdsall, K. (2001) *Sociology,* 4th edition. Cambridge: Polity Press.

Gieryn, T.F. (1983) 'Boundary work and the demarcation of science from non-science: strains and interests in the professional ideologies of scientists.' *American Sociological Review 48,* 6, 781–795.

Gieryn, T.F. (1995) 'Boundaries of science.' In S. Jasanoff, G.E. Markle, J.C. Petersen and T. Pinch (eds) *Handbook of Science and Technology Studies.* London: Sage.

Giles, H. and Coupland, N. (1991) *Language: Contexts and Consequences.* Pacific Grove, CA: Brooks/Cole Publishing Company.

Gilleard, C. and Higgs, P. (2000) *Cultures of Ageing: Self, Citizen and the Body.* Harlow: Prentice Hall.

Goffman, E. (1968) *Stigma: Notes on the Management of Spoiled Identity.* Harmondsworth: Penguin Books.

Graham, R. (2004) 'Cognitive citizenship: access to hip surgery for people with dementia.' *Health 8,* 3, 295–310.

Gubrium, J.F. (1987) 'Structuring and de-structuring the course of illness: the Alzheimer's disease experience.' *Sociology of Health and Illness 9,* 1–24.

Harris, P.B. (ed) (2002a) *The Person with Alzheimer's Disease: Pathways to Understanding the Experience.* Baltimore and London: Johns Hopkins University Press.

Harris, P.B. (2002b) 'The subjective experience of early on-set dementia: voices of the persons.' *Gerontologist 42,* Special Issue 1, 384.

Hulko, W. (2002) 'Making the links: social theories, experiences of people with dementia, and intersectionality.' In A. Leibing and L. Scheinkman (eds) *The Diversity of Alzheimer's Disease: Different Approaches and Contexts.* Rio de Janeiro, Brazil: CUCA-IPUB.

Huppert, F.A., Brayne, C. and O'Connor, D.W. (1994) *Dementia and Normal Aging.* Cambridge: Cambridge University Press.

Jenkins, R. (1991) 'Disability and social stratification.' *British Journal of Sociology 42,* 4, 557–580.

Kay, D.W.K. and Roth, M. (2002) 'Pathological correlates of dementia [letter].' *The Lancet 359,* 624–625.

Kirkwood, T. (1999) *Time of Our Lives: The Science of Human Ageing.* London: Weidenfeld and Nicolson.

Kitwood, T. (1997) *Dementia Reconsidered: The Person Comes First.* Buckingham: Open University Press.

Lash, S. and Urry, J. (1986) 'Dissolution of the social?' In M.L. Wardell and S.P. Turner (eds) *Sociological Theory in Transition.* London: Sage.

Laslett, P. (1977) 'The history of ageing and the aged.' In *Family Life and Illicit Love in Earlier Generations.* Cambridge: Cambridge University Press.

Lemert, E. (1964) 'Social structure, social control and deviation.' In M.B. Clinard (ed) *Anomie and Deviant Behaviour: A Discussion and Critique.* New York: Free Press.

Lyman, K.A. (1989) 'Bringing the social back in: a critique of the biomedicalisation of dementia.' *Gerontologist 29,* 5, 597–605.

Lyman, K.A. (1998) 'Living with Alzheimer's disease: the creation of meaning among persons with dementia.' *Journal of Clinical Ethics 9*, 1, 49–57.

Macrae, H. (1999) 'Managing courtesy stigma: the case of Alzheimer's disease.' *Sociology of Health and Illness 21*, 1, 54–70.

Manthorpe, J. (2000) 'Dementia in contemporary fiction and biography.' *Journal of Dementia Care 8*, 3, 35–37.

McGown, D. (1993) *Living in the Labyrinth*. New York: Delacorte Press.

Mead, G.H. (1934) *Mind, Self and Society*. Chicago: The University of Chicago Press.

Neuropathology Group of the Medical Research Council Cognitive Function and Ageing Study (MRC CFAS) (2001) 'Pathological correlates of late-onset dementia in a multicentre, community-based population in England and Wales.' *The Lancet 357*, 169–175.

Oliver, M. (1996) *Understanding Disability*. Basingstoke: Macmillan.

Phillipson, C. (1982) *Capitalism and the Construction of Old Age*. London: Macmillan.

Phillipson, C. (1998) *Reconstructing Old Age: New Agendas in Social Theory and Practice*. London: Sage.

Popper, K.R. (1961) *The Poverty of Historicism*. London: Routledge and Kegan Paul.

Post, S. (1995) *The Moral Challenge of Alzheimer's Disease*. Baltimore and London: The Johns Hopkins University Press.

Riley, M.W., Johnson, M. and Finer, A. (1972) *Ageing and Society: A Sociology of Age Stratification*. New York: Russel Sage Foundation.

Sabat, S.R. (2001) *The Experience of Alzheimer's Disease: Life Through a Tangled Veil*. Oxford: Blackwell.

Sawchuk, K.A. (1995) 'From gloom to boom: age, identity and target marketing.' In M. Featherstone and A. Wernick (eds) *Images of Aging: Cultural Representations of Later Life*. London: Routledge.

Sterin, G.J. (2002) 'Essay on a word: a lived experience of Alzheimer's disease.' *Dementia 1*, 1, 7–10.

Townsend, P. (1981) 'The structured dependency of the elderly: a creation of social policy in the twentieth century.' *Ageing and Society 1*, 5–28.

United Nations (2000) *The Ageing of the World's Population*. www.un.org/esa/socdev/ageing/agewpop.htm, accessed 10/04/2002.

Walker, A. (1980) 'The social creation of poverty and dependency in old age.' *Journal of Social Policy 9*, 59–75.

Walker, A. (1981) 'Towards a political economy of old age.' *Ageing and Society 1*, 73–94.

Zola, I.K. (1972) 'Medicine as an institution of social control.' *Sociological Review 20*, 4, 487–504.

CHAPTER 15

Social Science Perspectives on Dementia Research: Intersectionality

Wendy Hulko

Introduction

The aims of this chapter are to introduce the concept of intersectionality, highlight its relevance for social science research on dementia, and address methodological issues arising from a grounded theory study of dementia and intersectionality. This chapter is based on research that was in progress at the time of writing, and that was concerned with subjective experiences of dementia in later life, particularly the influence of one's social location on this life process. Explorations of the subjective realm of dementia are fairly recent (see Braudy Harris 2002; Downs 1997; Proctor 2001; Wilkinson 2002; Woods 2001), despite researchers having highlighted this gap well over a decade ago (Cotrell and Schulz 1993; Froggatt 1988; Lyman 1989). Moreover, this body of research is incomplete, as minimal attention has been paid to the influence of identity categories such as age, class, gender, 'race'[1] and ethnicity (Disman 1991; Downs 2000; Hulko 2002). Socio-cultural factors such as one's gender, 'racial', ethnic and class identity impact on one's world view and life course and are thus an important consideration in seeking to understand what it is like to live with dementia.

Despite the growing voices of people living with dementia, these have largely excluded the input and participation of people who belong to traditionally marginalised groups (Hulko 2002). We will not know whether and in what way an individual's unique, complex and intersecting identity shapes their experience of dementia until we include these questions in our research and ask them directly of the people whose lives we are studying. Moving away from selfhood and personhood into the realm of identity calls for an analysis of intersectionality – a metaphor for the entanglement and interaction of multiple and complex identity categories. If we are to move beyond narrow conceptions of personhood that are now claiming space alongside biomedical views of dementia, and for which credit is due to Tom Kitwood and his colleagues striving towards a 'new culture of dementia care' (see Kitwood 1990, 1997; Kitwood and Benson 1995; Kitwood and Bredin 1992), we must expand the epistemological and ontological bases of dementia research, embrace lessons from parallel knowledge traditions, and develop theory that is grounded in the voices of people experiencing this phenomenon. This chapter introduces a study that was designed to achieve these aims and uses it as a case study to highlight emerging issues for social science research in dementia. After an introduction to the concept of intersectionality, I present findings from the literature related to dementia and intersectionality, focusing on dementia theorising, subjective experiences of dementia, identity factors and social location. I then describe the research project, discuss methodological issues that have arisen and conclude with comments about the potential implications of a grounded theory of dementia and intersectionality, and key questions that have arisen from the study.

Intersectionality: meaning and use of this concept

As I have discussed elsewhere (Hulko 2002), intersectionality as a theoretical concept and analytical perspective has been used by scholars and activists in critical legal theory, feminism, anti-racism, and more recently social work and critical gerontology. Intersectionality is used to point out the reality that we are all holistic beings, inhabiting multiple and complex identities that should not be teased apart into separate units of analysis (Andersen and Hill Collins 2001; Bannerji 1995; Brah 2001; Dressel, Minkler and Yen 1997; Lorde 2001; Woodward 1997). Further, we each possess different degrees of oppression and privilege based on our relative positioning along axes of interlocking systems of oppression, such as racism, classism, sexism, ethnocentrism and ageism. Where each of us lies in relation to the centre and the margin (hooks 2000) – our social location – is determined by our identities, which are necessarily intersectional. Intersectionality is related to key sociological concepts such as identity, social location, subjectivity and the self, all of which have been a focus of intense interest within the dementia field in recent years. There are two approaches to the study of identity/subjectivity, with one approach seeing identity as 'fixed and trans-historical' (essentialism) and the other treating identity as 'fluid and contingent' (Woodward 1997). This study takes the latter approach, using the terms 'identity' and 'subjectivity' interchangeably, recognising that the former has a political meaning (Bannerji 1995) while the latter denotes status as a subject and signifies the coming to voice of oppressed peoples (Mama 1995).

'Intersectionality' and its corollary 'interlocking oppressions' have been applied to human rights claims/discrimination cases (OHRC 2001) in the critical race theory tradition (Crenshaw Williams 1989, 1994; Delgado 1995; Delgado and Stefancic 2001). However, this has not been accompanied by empirical research to date. Intersectionality may feel right and make sense intuitively as a way of thinking about our multiple selves, and may appear theoretically and politically attractive as it leads us away from fruitless attempts to find the ultimate oppression to which all others can be reduced. However, it needs to be bolstered by empirical research, a task made daunting by the fact that it is a very difficult concept to operationalise, and efforts to do so are rarely discussed (see Hulko 2003). Nevertheless, it represents an important development in thinking about identity and difference and could offer valuable insights for dementia research.

Knowledge to date about dementia theorising, subjective experiences, identity and social location

Given the dearth of literature specifically related to the topic of dementia and intersectionality, the literature review that I undertook for this project involved extensive reading in the substantive field of dementia, as well as sampling of material from related disciplines and parallel knowledge fields. I sought out knowledge about subjective experiences of dementia, as well as concepts, evidence and theories that could potentially assist in the development of a grounded theory of dementia and intersectionality. Since I have detailed elsewhere my findings related to dementia theorising and subjective experiences of dementia (Hulko 2002), I will summarise this material and then give an overview of the literature related to identity and social location.

Dementia theorising has been largely ontological in nature, focused on what dementia is or how it should be viewed, and thus the question of how dementia is experienced has been largely overlooked (Hulko 2002). The absence of phenomenological perspectives on dementia is an acknowledged gap in the literature and accounts for my attention to ontological theories of dementia in this review. The divergent and overlapping dementia theories that have been put forth to date see dementia as:

- a brain disease
- normal ageing
- a psycho-neurological condition
- a disability
- a mental health problem
- a social construction.

While this proliferation of theories is indicative of growing disaffection with the medical model (Bond 1992; Estes and Binney 1991; Lyman 1989; Robertson 1992), chiefly for its inability to adequately explain this phenomenon called dementia (see Leibing 2002), theories which address the social and environmental context of dementia have not been free of some of the limitations of their predecessors. The brain disease and normal ageing theories were the first explanatory theories of dementia put forth and have yet to be reconciled with one another, despite the fact that both are rooted in the biomedical paradigm. The psychological and sociological theories that followed did not alter the ontological course of dementia theorising in that they are not grounded in the voices and experiences of people living with dementia, nor do they take into consideration identity factors and social location. It appears that the next step should be to try to develop theory through the active engagement of people with dementia themselves, taking into consideration their socio-cultural context (Downs 2000).

In my search for information on subjective experiences of dementia, I reviewed personal accounts, narratives produced with the involvement of a supportive other, qualitative research studies, and stories posted on websites or available in hard copy for the purpose of raising public awareness (see Hulko 2002). I looked closely at who is telling these stories of dementia; what these stories tell; and whose voices are still silent/silenced. Then I asked myself how untold experiences might differ. I found that the 'typical' person with dementia in these published accounts was a middle-aged (40 to 60 years old), well-educated, white, married professional in the early stages of dementia, with strong religious or ideological beliefs, and a supportive family. The voices that are missing in the dementia literature are those of minority ethnic and racialised people, poor people, uneducated or minimally educated people, and lesbian/gay/bisexual/two-spirited people; and while the voices of older and disabled people do appear, this is certainly not a dominant feature. Identity was rarely treated as a salient variable in the literature and was certainly not viewed as multiple, complex and simultaneously expressed. When identity categories such as age, gender and ethnicity were mentioned at all, it was in a descriptive fashion in that any influence these factors might have on subjective experiences was not analysed. Yet despite this omission, through a close reading of the texts, I was able to discern class, gender, religion and age effects in the views and stories told by people living with dementia and found evidence of intersectional thinking on the part of the respondents. With regards to how untold stories might differ, a predominant theme in the literature was that of 'striving for normalcy', with normal being used to refer to life before/without dementia. This theme does not leave space for those who might have been striving for normalcy prior to a diagnosis of dementia or who reject societal definitions of normalcy.

From reviewing the literature on meanings of health, illness and disability cross-culturally; identity and oppression; 'race'/ethnicity and dementia; class, gender and dementia; and inequalities in later life, I garnered further insights that shaped this study. For example, conceptions of illness show similarities and differences across and within cultures and certain concepts are helpful to understanding how individuals make meaning of their experiences, including illness narratives (Kleinman 1988) and exploratory maps (Williams and Healy 2001). While insiders' perspectives such as these are valuable, they should be critically analysed, considering the temporal and socio-cultural context in which the teller lives and the tale is told. Researchers in turn need to design studies in a way that connections can be made between subjective meaning making (individual experiences) and the social forces that both support and impede these efforts (social structures), a longstanding problematic in sociology (Smith 1987).

Research on 'race'/ethnicity to date has focused on: comparative risk, incidence and prevalence rates for various racialised groups; challenges in assessment and diagnosis in a multicultural context; provision of services to minority ethnic and racialised people with dementia and their caregivers; caregiving among minority ethnic and racialised groups; and the meanings of dementia for certain minority ethnic and racialised groups. There is an obvious gap in that lived experiences of dementia have not been a concern for researchers interested in 'race'/ethnicity and dementia and, interestingly, many 'racial'/ethnic differences fall away when education is controlled for (Yeo 2001), a finding which indicates the entangled nature of identity categories.

Another factor that may prove to be the unspoken, yet most salient, variable in dementia research is class, and it may be that people belonging to the
upper class are more fearful of dementia (Hellebrandt 1980) because it represents more significant losses in terms of their social roles, while those from the
lower class are accustomed to dealing with adversity and dementia represents
one more challenge to overcome. Gender may prove to be significant in terms
of adherence to or liberation from gendered identities in the context of
dementia and the ways in which gender relations mediate experiences of
dementia for both men and women. It may be difficult, however, to ascertain
men's views of the influence of their gender as it seems that they are not accustomed to thinking of themselves in this way, unlike women who are said to
possess epistemic privilege (Whitehead 2001). This is akin to Du Bois' theory
of double consciousness (1953) which postulates that oppressed people,
being conscious of the dynamics of privilege and oppression and their own
relative positioning, are able to see both the privilege of their oppressors and
the way that efforts to sustain that privilege result in their own oppression.
Thus, it may be unfamiliar for white people to talk about the effect of their
'race' on their experiences, as most do not recognise their whiteness as having
an influence, particularly in terms of privilege.

It appears that social location has an influence in terms of people's
conceptualisations of their experiences and that privilege and oppression
need to be considered as dialectical, rather than oppositional (Bishop 2002;
Freire 2001). This means that we need to interrogate privilege as well as
oppression, as social life is relational and it is the same power dynamics shaping privilege as oppression, including the relative amount we each hold and
the meaning this has for our life experiences (Calasanti 1996). Several critical
gerontologists note the importance of looking at forms of oppression as interacting with one another in complex ways; and as rooted in processes of
domination and subordination; plus viewing marginalised peoples as having
strengths; and as actively resisting oppression (Blakemore 1989; Browne
1995; Calasanti 1996; Calasanti and Slevin 2001; Dressel 1991; Ginn and
Arber 1995; Gonyea 1994; Levy 1988; McMullin 2000; Minkler 1996; Victor 1991; Vincent 1995). A key concern arising from the literature on
intersectionality/interlocking oppressions, however, is that this is a difficult
concept to operationalise and thus there is a lack of empirical research to sub-
stantiate all the theorising and personal reflections. Trying to address this gap
clearly requires creativity and a willingness to take chances with one's
research design and data collection tools, particularly interview questions,
along with reflexivity in the field to follow possible leads, weave together

threads of meaning, and make connections between individual experiences and social structures. These are all lessons that apply to this project on dementia and intersectionality, which I will describe in the next section.

Grounded theory research into subjective experiences of dementia and intersectionality

It became apparent after a thorough review of the literature that this project could not be anything but exploratory in nature and qualitative in design, and that grounded theory methods (Charmaz 2000; Glaser 2001; Glaser and Strauss 1967; Strauss and Corbin 1998) could best address the research question – what the relationships are between older people's experiences of dementia and the intersections of 'race', ethnicity, class and gender. The research aims, which reflect the feminist, critical gerontology and anti-oppressive social work stance I brought to this project, were:

- to explore older people's experiences of living with a cognitive impairment, taking account of 'race', ethnicity, class, gender and their intersections and the dynamics of privilege and oppression

- to develop a substantive theory of older people's experiences of dementia and a formal theory of dementia and intersectionality, grounded in the voices and (inter)actions of older people with dementia

- to critically reflect on the research process, particularly the roles and effects on the researcher, the researched and the emerging theory, and the applicability and effectiveness of anti-oppressive research methods.

Using grounded theory meant that the research design would be emergent and this would require me to be reflective, reflexive and able to tolerate a degree of uncertainty. For example, the size and composition of the sample and the interview questions evolved throughout the course of the project, based on the results of the simultaneous collection and analysis of data and my reflections on the effectiveness of the methods I was using. The other grounded theory strategies I used were: two step data coding process; comparative methods; memo writing to construct conceptual analyses; sampling to refine emerging theoretical ideas; and integration of the theoretical framework (Charmaz 2000, pp.510–11). I was determined that this would apply from conception through completion in the classic grounded theory tradition (Glaser and Strauss 1967) and wanted to avoid a mistake noted in the literature (Glaser 2001; Strauss and Corbin 1994) whereby researchers claimed to have used a grounded theory approach when it is little more than inductive analysis. The generation of theory that is grounded in the data – not merely conceptual description – is the hallmark of grounded theory research (Glaser 2001) and 'all three aspects of inquiry (induction, deduction and verification) are absolutely essential' (Strauss 1987, p.12) in order to achieve this result. Through engaging in grounded theory, infusing it with anti-oppression sensibilities and reflecting on my experiences throughout, I hoped to add to these and other methodological debates about this popular and seemingly misunderstood method of research. The themes in the literature and the suggestions put forth for doing research with people with dementia, together with my own experience in dementia care and research, informed the design of this project.

My data collection tools included interviews, participant observation and photography with older people with dementia who ranged from multiply oppressed to multiply privileged, and focus groups with their significant others. I used conversation aids such as images of older people and third party questioning to increase both comfort and familiarity with the questions and to help to unlock subjectivity, and photographs of my research participants that I took at the observation sessions and in their homes, as well as family pictures that they shared with me, to stimulate thinking about life with memory problems. My sample evolved throughout the project in accordance with theoretical sampling (Glaser and Strauss 1967), and was comprised of older people with dementia in two different communities who were recruited through a local geriatrician and the Alzheimer's Society in one community, and a clinic for older people at an acute care hospital in the other. Over the course of a month, I would do three semi-structured interviews of 30 minutes to an hour and a half with a participant, interspersed with two observation sessions of about two hours at a setting or event of their choosing. The interview questions were designed to stimulate self-identification in terms of identity and social location and to evoke thoughts on living with memory problems. I used a Polaroid camera as I felt this would be more dementia-friendly than a digital camera or a 35 mm camera, primarily for the instantaneous photo developing, and the size and appearance of the photographs. As a result of this, I was able to speak with my participants about the events, people and objects captured on film at the time that they occurred and I could leave behind a record of the time that we spent together to serve as a memory aid for my next visit. I used a computer program to assist with the data analysis – N*VIVO – and once I became comfortable with its operation, it enabled me to organise all of the data collected and to perform functions such as linking documents, embedding visual data and memos, and modelling relationships (Lonkila 1995; Richards 2000). More details of my methods will be offered in the subsequent discussion of the methodological challenges I encountered.

Methodological challenges and attempts to address them

Several methodological challenges have arisen in the course of this research project on dementia and intersectionality and, while they are specific to this project on dementia and intersectionality, they offer insights for other research endeavours in dementia. In this section, I will raise the issues and describe my attempts to address them thus far.[2] The challenges I encountered relate to:

- configuring the sample
- translating sociological concepts
- describing the project
- designing interview questions
- being reflective and reflexive.

Configuring the sample

In configuring my sample, I had to resist the pull towards essentialism that seems to arise in research related to identity and difference. I knew that my participants, as a group, should represent various social locations, rather than different mathematical configurations of the variables of 'race', ethnicity, class and gender. However, I was not sure how to accomplish this so I played with different algebraic formulas in an effort to devise a 'diverse sample' and considered using Ragin's (1994) truth table method of quantifying data when researching diversity. I was able to reject this process of essentialising people with its ostensible goal of simplifying complexity/diversity once I came upon an alternate method that was more in line with my research aims and still resulted in a sufficiently diverse sample. My approach calls for the selection of people who lie at different points on the axes of oppression and privilege, based on their 'race', ethnicity, class and gender. In this way, similar/shared social locations, ranging from multiply privileged to multiply oppressed, rather than individual characteristics, form the basis upon which the sample is stratified. I was aided by a tool that is popular in anti-oppression workshops for graphically determining one's own social location. In this exercise, multiple axes of oppression and privilege are drawn in a form reminiscent of the spokes of a wheel and each is labelled with a different identity construct; that is, age, gender, class, sexual orientation, 'race', ethnicity, religion, (dis) ability, language, health status. The centre of the circle represents privilege and the outside represents oppression/marginalisation (see Hooks 2000). The task is to situate oneself on each of these axes in relation to the margin and the centre and, through doing so, to become (more) conscious of the degree of privilege and oppression one owns and which makes the everyday world problematic (Smith 1987), more so for some than for others. I did not plan to make these diagrams with my participants; rather I used the socio-demographic information I was given to construct a diagram for each participant and then located each of them along a continuum from multiply oppressed to multiply privileged. This process necessarily took place over the course of the project as people entered the project at different points and I assessed the composition of my sample.

Translating sociological concepts

The second challenge I had to deal with on an ongoing basis was in the translation of sociological concepts. Theoretical questions had to be translated to research questions, and then turned into interview questions that could be expressed in everyday language. The questions asked of participants had to be understandable and respectful at the same time, while still derivative of the original theoretical concepts to enable back translation. For example, the title of my thesis 'Dementia and intersectionality: exploring the experiences of older people with dementia and their significant others' became 'How does who you are as a person shape living with memory problems?' on the information leaflets and consent forms. To ensure that my materials would be understandable to older people with memory problems, I checked the readability statistics in MS Word and edited these documents repeatedly until the information leaflet was at a grade four level and ratio of 86/100 for reading ease, and the consent form was at a grade five level and ratio of 76/100 for reading ease. The standard is a grade seven to eight level with a ratio of 60–70/100 for reading ease. Sociological concepts can be complex and since these are not often the terms we use to describe ourselves, it was very difficult to explain this research in written and verbal form. The following excerpt from the information leaflet for research participants lists factors upon which people differ or how we are all unique and represents my attempt to translate gender, ethnicity, 'race' and class into plain language:

- whether we are a man or a woman
- the languages we speak, food we eat and clothes we wear
- where we come from
- how old we are
- how other people see us
- the schooling, jobs and money we have or had
- how easy or hard life is for us.

'Race' is not easily identifiable in this list; the language I have used could be thought to refer to age or disability. This probably has more to do with my own discomfort over using certain words or phrases, such as skin colour, that may be more descriptive yet indicate acceptance of the ideology of racial differences.

Describing the project

Describing the project was a concern not only for my interactions with research participants, but also with each of the interpreters that I worked with and all the gatekeepers, meaning 'those individuals in an organisation who have the power to grant or withhold access to people or situations for the purposes of research' (Burgess 1984, p.48). The gatekeepers I had to pass through in order to speak with older people with dementia included the research director and research committee, programme manager, geriatricians, professional and administrative staff, and public affairs department at one recruiting site; the Alzheimer's Society executive director and support counsellors, and a geriatrician and administrative staff at the other site; the people in charge at the various observation settings; and the significant others in both locations in the case of those people whom I was told not to contact directly. I demonstrated my legitimacy/credentials in order to gain access to research participants and to build rapport with gatekeepers, yet essentially had little control over which of their clients they chose to refer to me. At first, most gatekeepers interpreted my research as being solely about minority ethnic and racialised people – the Other – and tended to place greater emphasis on language and 'race'/ethnicity than either gender or class. As the inclusion of privileged people is equally as important in seeking to understand the dynamics of privilege and oppression (Calasanti and Slevin 2001; Lee 1993) and hence was critical for my study, I had to continually explain to the gatekeepers what I was attempting to do, why, and how they could help me, while being attentive to any misinterpretations that might have been transmitted to potential participants. For example, one recruiting site left me a message that they had 'one for race, one for race and class, and one for ethnicity'. I interpreted this as meaning these people were marginalised on these grounds and privileged on the basis of the factors not mentioned, and clarified the next time we talked that each of us has a gender, class, 'race' and ethnicity.

Designing interview questions

The challenges in designing the interview questions relate to my interest in facilitating self-identification and the expression of subjectivity on the part of my research participants. This was in the hopes of avoiding mislabelling people or placing too great or too little importance on an aspect of their identity. To try and achieve this goal, I posed general questions such as 'tell me some important things about yourself'; 'when you think of yourself, what image comes to mind?'; and 'how would other people describe you?'. These questions did not elicit the responses I was hoping for at the beginning of my research as, more often than not, participants referred to personality characteristics. I realised that I had to be more direct with my questioning, as in 'what is it like to be an old Filipina woman?'. I used images of older people who were diversified by ethnicity, 'race', class and gender and asked questions about the people in the pictures such as 'what do you think of him/her?'; 'who has the best/worst deal in life?'; and 'who is the most/least like you?'. I had difficulty overcoming my own reservations about being insensitive or too personal and using language that I was not comfortable with such as 'old' or asking questions of a black man that seemed self-evident such as 'so why is he a brother?' in reference to a picture of another black man.

Being reflective and reflexive

The last challenge is that of being both reflective and reflexive, which essentially means 'being on' at all times, continually analysing and responding to insights derived from the research process. Reflection represents the critical introspection the researcher undergoes and reflexivity the action that flows from this; the latter being akin to 'praxis' in Marxist terms (see Kirby and McKenna 1989). These terms are often conflated in methodological discussions, however, with researchers referring to the importance of reflexivity in the sense of documenting one's reactions to the research and situating oneself in the research process, yet not giving any evidence of their methods having been modified on the basis of these reflections. For this project, I carried a reflective journal with me in which I recorded thoughts on the research process; made notes on most encounters, particularly the initial one which was the information and consent meeting; introduced new questions and/or put aside the pictures if they didn't appear to be achieving the desired result; developed an interview guide prior to each encounter based on my analysis to date; and consulted with peers about my techniques and results. Despite all of these efforts, I feel that I could have been even more reflexive if I had the time and concentration to thoroughly reflect, and the freedom from institutional expectations or constraints, such as those imposed by the recruiting site, ethical review committee and funders.

Conclusion: possible implications and key questions

At the time of this writing, the data collection and analysis was still in progress and therefore possible implications are tentative. A grounded theory of dementia and intersectionality could further our understandings of lived experiences of dementia in later life, and address the socio-cultural context of dementia. It may well lead to further questions about how to design and deliver services that are based on the desires of users, rather than on the opinions of providers about what older people with dementia need; and it could raise the controversial issue as to whether we should be intervening in their lives at all. As this research project drew on parallel knowledge traditions and crossed disciplinary boundaries, the findings are likely to have implications for several fields of study and various disciplines; and the implications could be for any level of scholarly activity such as theory, research, policy and practice. As the potential audience is wide and the research–policy–practice interface important to me, I plan to disseminate the findings widely, which will necessarily entail publishing in multiple genres (DeVault 1999; Fine *et al.* 2000) to ensure that all those who may benefit from having the information have access to it (Kirby and McKenna 1989). For my research participants, I committed to preparing a summary of one to two pages in an accessible format and to sharing this information with them verbally, in a group format or one-on-one sessions. Some dementia researchers might question the purpose and utility of sharing results with participants as the nature of their cognitive impairment may preclude any understanding of that which is presented to them. Yet, as Elaine Robinson (2002) writes of her experience taking part in research, 'it would be very disheartening for us to spend our time taking part in interviews or providing written material only to find that we never hear from those conducting the research' (p.106). I only hope that the emerging theory makes sense to the people upon whose experiences it is based and that it can be presented to them and others in an accessible format that will empower, rather than alienate. If it does not make sense, then does their cognitive impairment impede their ability to understand or has the researcher not accurately reflected their perspectives and experiences? This is a question that researchers are forced to grapple with in seeking to involve participants meaningfully. Do participants need to talk about themselves as intersectional beings or is this the lens and the methodology that the researcher brings to the project? Working with the concept of intersectionality can be cognitively demanding due to its complexity and may require a politically conscious subject. If that is the case, we may set ourselves up for failure if we try to move beyond our analytical frame as researchers using an intersectional perspective and look for evidence of intersectional thinking in the words and actions of our participants. These are some key questions that have arisen to date and for which it is hoped some answers may emerge. Through presenting this work in progress as a case study and detailing the methodological issues that have arisen in working with the concept of intersectionality, perhaps other researchers may encounter useful insights for their own work and choose to grapple with these and other complex questions.

Notes

1   I use 'race' in quotation marks and racialised people (Fanon 1963) to denote that I subscribe to the view that race is socially constructed (see Haney López 1995). Moreover, it should remain an important focus of sociological analysis as long as the attributes ascribed to different 'races' and the resulting hierarchies remain in existence, shaping our experiences of privilege and oppression (see Crenshaw Williams 1994).

2   These ideas were developed further in a conference paper given after this chapter was written (Hulko 2003).

References

Andersen, M.L. and Hill Collins, P. (eds) (2001) *Race, Class, and Gender: An Anthology*, 4th edition. Belmont: Wadsworth.

Bannerji, H. (1995) 'The passion of naming: identity, difference and politics of class.' *Thinking Through: Essays on Feminism, Marxism, and Anti-racism*. Toronto: Women's Press.

Bishop, A. (2002) *Becoming an Ally: Breaking the Cycle of Oppression in People*, 2nd edition. London and New York: Zed Books; Halifax: Fernwood Publishing.

Blakemore, K. (1989) 'Does age matter? The case of old age in minority ethnic groups.' In B. Bytheway, T. Keil, P. Allatt and A. Bryman (eds) *Becoming and Being Old: Sociological Approaches to Later Life*. London: Sage.

Bond, J. (1992) 'The medicalisation of dementia.' *Journal of Aging Studies 6*, 397–403.

Brah, A. (2001) 'Difference, diversity, differentiation.' In K. Bhavnani (ed) *Feminism and 'Race'*. Oxford: Oxford University Press.

Braudy Harris, P. (ed) (2002) *The Person with Alzheimer's Disease: Pathways to Understanding the Experience*. Baltimore, MD: Johns Hopkins University Press.

Browne, C. (1995) 'A feminist life span perspective on ageing.' In N. Van Den Bergh (ed) *Feminist Practice in the 21st Century*. Washington: NASW Press.

Burgess, R.G. (1984) 'Starting research and gaining access.' *In the Field: An Introduction to Field Research*. London: Routledge.

Calasanti, T. (1996) 'Incorporating diversity: meaning, levels of research, and implications for theory.' *The Gerontologist 36*, 2, 147–156.

Calasanti, T.M. and Slevin, K.F. (2001) *Gender, Social Inequalities, and Aging*. Walnut Creek, CA: Altamira Press.

Charmaz, K. (2000) 'Grounded theory: objectivist and constructivist methods.' In N.K. Denzin and Y.S. Lincoln (eds) *Handbook of Qualitative Research*, 2nd edition. Thousand Oaks, CA: Sage.

Cotrell, V. and Schulz, R. (1993) 'The perspective of the person with Alzheimer's Disease: a neglected dimension of dementia research.' *The Gerontologist 33*, 2, 205–211.

Crenshaw Williams, K. (1989) 'Demarginalising the intersection of race and sex: a Black Feminist critique of anti-discrimination doctrine, feminist theory and antiracist politics.' *University of Chicago Legal Forum*.

Crenshaw Williams, K. (1994) 'Mapping the margins: intersectionality, identity politics, and violence against women of colour.' In M. Fineman and R. Mykitiuk (eds) *The Public Nature of Private Violence*. New York: Routledge.

Delgado, R. (ed) (1995) *Critical Race Theory: The Cutting Edge*. Philadelphia: Temple University Press.

Delgado, R. and Stefancic, J. (2001) *Critical Race Theory: An Introduction*. New York: New York University Press.

DeVault, M.L. (1999) *Liberating Method: Feminism and Social Research*. Philadelphia: Temple University Press.

Disman, M. (1991) 'The subjective experience of Alzheimer's disease: a socio-cultural perspective.' *The American Journal of Alzheimer's Care and Related Disorders and Research 6*, 3, 30–34.

Downs, M. (1997) 'The emergence of the person in dementia research.' *Ageing and Society 17*, 597–607.

Downs, M. (2000) 'Dementia in a socio-cultural context: an idea whose time has come.' *Ageing and Society 20*, 369–375.

Dressel, P. (1991) 'Gender, race and class: beyond the feminisation of poverty in later life.' In M. Minkler and C. Estes (eds) *Critical Perspectives on Aging: The Political and Moral Economy of Growing Old*. Amityville, NY: Baywood.

Dressel, P., Minkler, M. and Yen, I. (1997) 'Gender, race, class, and ageing: advances and opportunities.' *International Journal of Health Services 27*, 4, 579–600.

Du Bois, W.E.B. (1953) *The Souls of Black Folk.* New York: Fawcett.

Estes, C. and Binney, E. (1991) 'The biomedicalization of ageing: dangers and dilemmas.' In M. Minkler and C. Estes (eds) *Critical Perspectives on Aging: The Political and Moral Economy of Growing Old.* Amityville, NY: Baywood.

Fanon, F. (1963) *The Wretched of the Earth.* London: Penguin.

Fine, M., Weis, L., Weseen, S. and Wong, L. (2000) 'For whom? Qualitative research, representations and social responsibilities.' In N.K. Denzin and Y.S. Lincoln (eds) *Handbook of Qualitative Research,* 2nd edition. Thousand Oaks, CA: Sage.

Freire, P. (2001) *Pedagogy of the Oppressed, 30th Anniversary Edition.* New York: Continuum.

Froggatt, A. (1988) 'Self-awareness in early dementia.' In B. Gearing, M. Johnson and T. Heller (eds) *Mental Health Problems in Old Age: A Reader.* Chichester: John Wiley and Sons.

Ginn, J. and Arber, S. (1995) '"Only connect": Gender relations and ageing.' In S. Arber and J. Ginn (eds) *Connecting Gender and Ageing: A Sociological Approach.* Buckingham: Open University Press.

Glaser, B.G. (2001) *The Grounded Theory Perspective: Conceptualisation Contrasted with Description.* Mill Valley, CA: Sociology Press.

Glaser, B.G. and Strauss, A.L. (1967) *The Discovery of Grounded Theory: Strategies for Qualitative Research.* New York: Aldine.

Gonyea, J.G. (1994) 'The paradox of the advantaged elder and the feminisation of poverty.' *Social Work 39*, 1, 35–41.

Haney López, I.F. (1995) 'The social construction of race.' In R. Delgado (ed) *Critical Race Theory: The Cutting Edge.* Philadelphia: Temple University Press.

Hellebrandt, F. (1980) 'Aging among the advantaged: a new look at the stereotype of the elderly.' *The Gerontologist 20*, 4, 404–417.

hooks, b. (2000) *Feminist Theory: From Margin to Center,* 2nd edition. Cambridge: South End Press.

Hulko, W. (2002) 'Making the links: social theories, experiences of people with dementia and intersectionality.' In A. Leibing and L. Scheinkman (eds) *The Diversity of Alzheimer's Disease: Different Approaches and Contexts.* Rio de Janeiro: CUCA-IPUB.

Hulko, W. (2003) 'Operationalising "intersectionality" in research with older people with dementia.' *Canadian Association of Schools of Social Work Conference,* Halifax, Canada, June.

Kirby, S. and McKenna, K. (1989) *Experience, Research, Social Change: Methods from the Margins.* Toronto: Garamond Press.

Kitwood, T. (1990) 'The dialectics of dementia: with particular reference to Alzheimer's Disease.' *Ageing and Society 10*, 177–196.

Kitwood, T. (1997) *Dementia Reconsidered: The Person Comes First.* Buckingham: Open University Press.

Kitwood, T. and Benson, S. (1995) *The New Culture of Dementia Care.* London: Hawker.

Kitwood, T. and Bredin, K. (1992) 'Towards a theory of dementia care: person-hood and well-being.' *Ageing and Society 12*, 269–287.

Kleinman, A. (1988) *The Illness Narratives: Suffering, Healing and the Human Condition.* New York: Basic Books.

Lee, R.M. (1993) 'The access issue in research on sensitive topics.' *Doing Research on Sensitive Topics.* London: Sage.

Leibing, A. (2002) 'Ideology and biology: some remarks on Alzheimer's Disease, genes, and risk in different populations.' In A. Leibing and L. Scheinkman (eds) *The Diversity of Alzheimer's Disease: Different Approaches and Contexts.* Rio de Janeiro: CUCA-IPUB.

Levy, J. (1988) 'Intersections of gender and ageing.' *The Sociological Quarterly 29,* 4, 479–486.

Lonkila, M. (1995) 'Grounded theory as an emerging paradigm for computer-assisted qualitative data analysis.' In U. Kelle (ed) *Computer-Aided Qualitative Data Analysis: Theory, Methods and Practice.* London: Sage.

Lorde, A. (2001) 'Age, race, class, and sex: women redefining difference.' In M.L. Andersen and P. Hill Collins (eds) *Race, Class, and Gender: An Anthology,* 4th edition. Belmont: Wadsworth.

Lyman, K. (1989) 'Bringing the social back in: a critique of the biomedicalization of dementia.' *The Gerontologist 29,* 5, 597–605.

Mama, A. (1995) *Beyond the Masks: Race, Gender and Subjectivity.* London: Routledge.

McMullin, J. (2000) 'Diversity and the state of sociological ageing theory.' *The Gerontologist 40,* 5, 517–530.

Minkler, M. (1996) 'Critical perspectives on ageing: new challenges for gerontology.' *Ageing and Society 16,* 467–487.

Ontario Human Rights Commission (OHRC) (2001) *An Intersectional Approach to Discrimination: Addressing Multiple Grounds in Human Rights Claims.* Toronto: Ontario Human Rights Commission.

Proctor, G. (2001) 'Listening to older women with dementia: relationships, voices and power.' *Disability and Society 16,* 3, 361–376.

Ragin, C. (1994) 'Using comparative methods to study diversity.' *Constructing Social Research.* Thousand Oaks, CA: Pine Forge Press.

Richards, L. (2000) *Using NVivo in Qualitative Research,* 2nd edition. Bundoora, Victoria: QSR International.

Robertson, A. (1990) 'The politics of Alzheimer's disease: a case study in apocalyptic demography.' *International Journal of Health Services 20,* 3, 429–442.

Robinson, E. (2002) 'Should people with Alzheimer's disease take part in research?' In H. Wilkinson (ed) *The Perspectives of People with Dementia: Research Methods and Motivations.* London: Jessica Kingsley Publishers.

Smith, D.E. (1987) *The Everyday World as Problematic: A Feminist Sociology.* Toronto: University of Toronto Press.

Strauss, A.L. (1987) *Qualitative Analysis for Social Scientists.* Cambridge, MA: Cambridge University Press.

Strauss, A. and Corbin, J. (1994) 'Grounded theory methodology: an overview.' In N.K. Denzin and Y.S. Lincoln (eds) *Handbook of Qualitative Research.* Newbury Park, CA: Sage.

Strauss, A. and Corbin, J. (1998) *Basics of Qualitative Research: Techniques and Procedures for Developing Grounded Theory*, 2nd edition. Thousand Oaks, CA: Sage.

Victor, C.R. (1991) 'Continuity or change: inequalities in health in later life.' *Ageing and Society 11*, 1, 23–39.

Vincent, J.A. (1995) *Inequality and Old Age.* London: UCL Press Ltd.

Whitehead, S.M. (2001) 'Man: the invisible gendered subject?' In S.M. Whitehead and F.J. Barrett (ed) *The Masculinities Reader.* Cambridge: Polity Press.

Wilkinson, H. (2002) 'Including people with dementia in research: methods and motivations.' In H. Wilkinson (ed) *The Perspectives of People with Dementia: Research Methods and Motivations.* London: Jessica Kingsley Publishers.

Williams, B. and Healy, D. (2001) 'Perceptions of illness causation among new referrals to a community mental health team: "explanatory model" or "exploratory map".' *Social Science and Medicine 53*, 4, 465–476.

Woods, B. (2001) 'Discovering the person with Alzheimer's disease: cognitive, emotional and behavioural aspects.' *Aging and Mental Health 5*, Supplement 1, S7–S16.

Woodward, K. (1997) 'Introduction.' In K. Woodward (ed) *Identity and Difference.* London: Sage.

Yeo, G. (2001) 'Ethnicity and dementia.' *Journal of the American Geriatric Society 49*, 10, 1393–1394.

CHAPTER 16

Dementia and Social Inclusion: The Way Forward

Caroline Cantley and Alison Bowes

Introduction

In this final chapter, we outline what we have learnt about the impact of social exclusion on people with dementia and their families, we draw together the processes that have been identified throughout this book as variously contributing to the social exclusion of people with dementia, and we summarise some of the suggestions that have been made for service developments to promote social inclusion. This chapter ends by discussing some of the fundamental issues and challenges that in future we will have to address if we are to create a society that truly includes people with dementia and their families.

Experiences and processes of social exclusion

Burden and Hamm (2000, p.184) suggest:

> Social exclusion can usefully be thought of as existing when groups of people are unable to achieve what are viewed as 'normal' levels of social acceptance and participation. This usually involves the lack of one or more of the following:
>
> • accepted levels of material well-being and of social benefits
> • commonly held legal and civil rights
> • a positive estimation of social status and identity.

Throughout this book we have seen how people with dementia experience social exclusion in different ways, at different times and to different degrees.

Perhaps most obviously, people with dementia experience social exclusion as physical restriction or segregation as a result of disabling environments and the 'batching' of people with similar needs by services such as day centres and care homes. But the social exclusion of people with dementia is much more pervasive than that. People with dementia experience social isolation from community and family life in a variety of other ways. They may have limited opportunities for meaningful occupation, for leisure activities, for artistic expression and for enjoyment of the arts. They may have difficulty maintaining contact with a faith community and as a result lack spiritual support and have limited opportunities for spiritual expression. Access to the knowledge and information that they need to plan and live their lives as fully as possible may be limited. They often experience services as difficult to access and as offering limited options in the extent of support available and in the type of lifestyles they will support. Exclusion has an impact on the self. People with dementia experience feelings of embarrassment and stigma, their sense of self and self-esteem is negatively affected, and they experience loss of dignity, stress and distress.

Social exclusion for people with dementia means that they are disempowered in a variety of ways. They have limited choice and control over their own lives, they may have difficulty participating in the decisions that affect their lives and ultimately their fundamental rights as citizens and human beings may be infringed. All these experiences and processes have been explored in the book.

Many of the contributors consider people with dementia in the context of wider social processes, and identify ways in which these can promote social exclusion. Bell for example argues that as everyone in modern society increasingly 'bowls alone', community appears to weaken, and stocks of social capital diminish, especially for those already marginalised. He suggests that issues of citizenship and inclusion present fundamental challenges for all, and that these are especially pressing where people already socially excluded are concerned.

Bell's theme of community resources and social capital also emerges in Innes and Sherlock's work on rural areas. While they warn against the dangers of assuming an idealised rurality, they nevertheless suggest that quality of life in rural areas is generally better as rural isolation obliges people to co-operate more fully with one another, mitigating against exclusionary processes. Similarly, Dilworth-Anderson's work highlights the significance of community co-operation and identification for the well-being of family caregivers.

Cobban's work on home care staff identifies their low status, which contrasts with their importance to the greater emphasis on care at home espoused by policy makers and service developers. Like people with dementia, care staff experience social exclusion, and this has an impact on the quality of care and support they are able to provide.

Marginalisation of people with dementia appears to be especially strong when they are dying. Cox and Watchman note that recent research and service development concerned with dying, including palliative care, has failed to deal with the particular issues presented by people with dementia, who may not easily respond to the organisational demands and structures put in place to enable 'good deaths'. Their work draws attention to exclusionary processes of stereotyping, whereby for example people with dementia's expressions of pain are not recognised.

Stereotyping is evident in Archibald's demonstration that people with dementia are not free to behave as they wish in their homes (in this case, residential care), being infantilised and having their behaviour explained away as a result of purported incapability.

In residential care contexts, lack of community, processes of marginalisation and stereotyping are shown to prevail in many cases. Müller-Hergl's explanation for the 'power fights' over faeces he identified in residential care settings lies in the lack of attention to building and sustaining social relationships. Similarly, Bruce illustrates how staff may stereotype people who have the impairment of dementia, interacting with them on the basis of these stereotypes rather than as individuals. She demonstrates that dementia and those who have it may be considered problematic in group-living contexts. People with dementia whose behaviour changes may find themselves removed from current living arrangements to more controlling alternatives, considered more suited to their condition – again, she suggests that little effort is put into work on social relationships, effective communication and interaction.

An important element in processes of exclusion is the tendency to see people with dementia primarily as service users, rather than as participants and stakeholders in ordinary social life. Manthorpe's discussion of risk identifies that, in the cases of people with dementia, assessment of risk presents particularly acute dilemmas, especially in terms of balancing consideration of risks with consideration of people's civil rights and their rights to self-determination. There is a tendency for perceptions of high risk to dominate, and for the care planning and provision process to over-ride people's own rights and desires. McColgan's account of 'nursing home culture' makes similar points, illustrating the reinforcement of exclusionary processes that can occur when the imperatives of the service over-ride those of the individual. Craig and Killick identify the silencing of people with dementia in hospital wards in which cleanliness, tidiness, white paint and white linen maintain the sanitised environment preferred by the institution.

Thus for people with dementia, disempowerment and exclusion come about through a range of interconnected factors and processes. These occur at all levels, from the collective ideological and cultural through to the interpersonal and psychological.

A range of cultural factors create social boundaries that distinguish people with dementia as being different, undesirable and stigmatised. The significance and status that Western culture accords rationality and cognitive competence is identified as one of the main factors contributing to the social exclusion of people with dementia. People with dementia may transgress, or be assumed to transgress, social expectations and norms especially in relation to social 'taboos', making public matters that are deemed to be properly 'private' in nature. Negative cultural assumptions about people with dementia are reinforced through the media where, despite an increasing profile for dementia, images remain primarily negative with very limited material that supports more socially inclusive visions.

The medical model's focus on people with dementia as being primarily 'patients' who embody a disease has contributed to exclusion. This ideological domination, reinforced through the institutions of medicine, has been to the detriment of other ideas such as understandings of personhood and how this can be nurtured and social disability models that emphasise the part that other people and social institutions play in creating the 'disability' that people with dementia experience.

Within Western capitalist society, people with dementia are often considered 'structurally dependent' because they are in large part older people who are no longer part of the workforce. People with dementia are frequently portrayed as an economic 'burden', who do not make positive contributions to society. Such portrayals feed negative stereotypes.

Power relationships within health and social care organisations can result in people with dementia experiencing services that are inadequately resourced and in which personnel have negative attitudes to their care. This reflects many of the wider social factors discussed above but also the low priority and status attached to dementia care by commissioning and providing organisations and by the professions. Staff involved in dementia services themselves are often low paid, female workers whose experience at work reflects their more general low social status and disempowerment. Even among the professions, staff in dementia services are generally deemed to be of lower status than their peers in other fields. These factors are compounded by under-investment in the development of dementia care skills in many services resulting in poor quality care and staff who feel undervalued and inadequately supported.

Exclusion from social participation and decreased social engagement often accompany older age and physical and mental frailty and restrict social interaction of and with people with dementia. Stereotyping promotes a notion of social incompetence for people with dementia and can operate at an interpersonal level to limit engagement with them. The condition, rather than the person, comes to dominate.

At an emotional or psychological level, responding to people with dementia frequently involves dealing with 'difficult issues' such as loss, death, sex and incontinence that evoke widespread and deep-seated emotional reactions of fear, guilt and shame. In such circumstances, emphasis on the condition rather than the person can apparently license a failure to respond effectively.

An inclusive future

A central aim of the book has been to examine what can and should be done to address the profound social exclusion of people with dementia, which extends to those who care for them. The contributors have identified many possible ways forward. We summarise these below in relation to: values; service development; and theory and research.

Values

Many contributors have, explicitly and implicitly, shown that greater social inclusion of people with dementia is predicated on value commitments. We can summarise the essence of the value stance required under the headings: personhood; relationship; and citizenship.

First, valuing the 'personhood' of each individual with dementia requires holistic approaches that reject too narrow a focus on cognitive abilities and that recognise the emotional, social, spiritual and artistic dimensions of the person. The emphasis on 'personhood' has been strong throughout the book, and is particularly exemplified by McColgan's observations on social competence and interaction and Cheston's account of the importance of listening to people with dementia's own reflections on their experiences. When attention is paid to these views and experiences, for example, people can be genuinely supported in the difficulties that a diagnosis of dementia may bring.

Second, valuing 'relationship' with people with dementia means that we must move away from narrow concerns about dependency and recognise the importance of interdependence and reciprocity. This involves enhancing 'mutuality' (Sapey 2001) and generating a sense of shared humanity founded on the spiritual and other benefits that those of us without dementia, as well as those with dementia, can gain from being with, and caring for and about, others. Bell and Dilworth-Anderson consider these issues at the level of community, and McColgan, Cheston, Craig and Killick look at interactive contexts in a range of institutional settings. Cobban explores relationships between home care workers and people with dementia. All stress that highlighting the social competencies and identities of people with dementia offers ways of challenging prevailing stereotypes.

Third, valuing citizenship means that we must have a commitment to social inclusion based on promoting ordinary living, ensuring that people with dementia retain as much choice and control as possible, and securing people's rights. Bond, Corner and Graham suggest the usefulness of the concept of 'cognitive citizenship' for drawing attention to ways in which these aims can be addressed. In residential care (Archibald, Bruce, McColgan, Müller-Hergl) the concept promotes challenge to exclusionary thinking and practice and in community-based services (Cobban, Manthorpe) it can support thinking about the exercise of rights balanced with assessments of risk. In wider community relations (Bell, Dilworth-Anderson, Innes and Sherlock), the concept draws attention to inclusionary processes permitting its exercise such as effective interaction and shared cultural norms and practices.

Service development

There are three main strands in the suggestions that contributors have made for service development to promote greater social inclusion of people with dementia.

First, services need to be more person centred and responsive to individual needs, circumstances and preferences. This requires services to be culturally sensitive to people from different social, economic, ethnic or faith communities. Hulko argues that people with dementia are as diverse in these respects as the whole population, and Dilworth-Anderson demonstrates the value of a culturally responsive community environment for family caregivers. Services must support and enhance individual identity, for example through meaningful occupation and access to the arts in their various forms as Craig and Killick's work exemplifies. The process requires developing innovative approaches to relating to people with dementia and hearing their voices, for example using non-verbal forms of communication, sensitive observation and engagement in the arts. Archibald's emphasis on the need to take seriously the sexuality of people with dementia, Cheston's emphasis on the need to facilitate voice and listen to people with dementia, Craig and Killick's work with the arts, and Müller-Hergl's stress on the need to build and sustain social relationships are all pertinent here.

Second, if service development is to promote inclusion, much greater investment is needed in staff support and development. In particular, it is essential: that staff in generic services are trained to respond appropriately to people with dementia who are using services for reasons other than their dementia; that dementia service providers recognise the centrality of the frontline staff who have extended and often long-term interaction with people with dementia; that staff in dementia services have training that includes input on how to deal with those aspects of care and support where changes in practice can prevent or reduce social exclusion. The impact that both negative and positive practices of frontline staff can have in residential care is clearly exemplified in Bruce, McColgan and Müller-Hergl's work.

Third, it has been argued that there is a need for further development of specialist services, for example in housing, home care, and care homes. It is also argued that there is a need for extending the availability of dementia specialist workers who can support staff in more generic services in responding better to the needs of people with dementia and enabling them to remain users of 'mainstream' services for longer. Cobban's suggestions for the potential role of specialist dementia workers both in directly providing services and in teaching others, both generic and specialist, to do so offer a potential way to improve this aspect. Similarly, Cox and Watchman reveal marked deficiencies of expertise in palliative care for people with dementia. Manthorpe's discussion of risk draws attention to ways in which the specialist consideration of issues in risk assessment for people with dementia can contribute to a wider process of reflection and a more general improvement in services for all categories of user.

Theory and research

From the foregoing discussions, we can draw a number of conclusions about how we can develop theory and research that will better address issues of social inclusion for people with dementia.

First, we need to address specific gaps in our knowledge, for example by undertaking research that can help us to understand better the diversity of experiences of living with dementia and the mechanisms and processes that lead to isolation and social exclusion of people with dementia and their families. Hulko's work in particular demonstrates the complexity of diversity, emphasising that this is best conceptualised in terms of multiple privilege versus multiple exclusion, rather than perpetuating an emphasis on one exclusionary factor, such as ethnicity or class, at the expense of others.

Second, there is the issue of how people with dementia can be involved in the processes of research and the development of theory. Several contributors have discussed research methodologies that ensure the perspectives of people with dementia are central and that they are obtained in participative ways rather than by treating people with dementia as passive 'respondents'. Cheston, Hulko, Innes and Sherlock, Craig and Killick and McColgan in particular have identified inclusive ways of conducting research, continuing the developing emphasis on this approach (Wilkinson 2002).

Third, it is important to ensure that dementia research and theory is not marginalised within academia. The advancement of our knowledge about people with dementia cannot happen in isolation. It must take place in the context of much broader developments in theory and research across a range of traditional academic disciplines and more applied interdisciplinary fields of study such as gerontology, family and community, mental health, and organisation and management studies. The need to maintain an interdisciplinary approach is exemplified in general terms by the diverse backgrounds of our contributors. In particular, Bond, Corner and Graham identify ways in which a range of sociological perspectives can be brought to bear on our understanding of the social position and experiences of people with dementia. Similarly, Hulko's work applies the concept of intersectionality to people with dementia, linking her discussion with work on diversity. Bradbury, Ballard and Fairbairn, working from a medical field, emphasise the need to revisit medical insights and to address questions which are central for people with dementia, but which have been recently marginalised within medical debates.

Issues and challenges

We have made the point above that discussion of exclusion needs to be conceptually contextualised. We therefore end by drawing on ideas and experiences of promoting social inclusion in related areas to identify some of the fundamental issues and challenges that we face if we are serious about an inclusive future for people with dementia.

Difference and commonality

Exploration of different facets of the experiences that people with dementia and their families have of being socially excluded has demonstrated how there are differences, in the sense of dissimilarities, between people with dementia and others, and also within the population of people with dementia. Recognising such differences is important if we are to understand and relate to the full range of life experiences of people with dementia. Some differences are clearly positive and easily celebrated. However, the central thesis of this book has been that, for most people with dementia, difference involves disadvantage and social exclusion.

We have seen how people with dementia in general experience aspects of social exclusion and how specific groups are further excluded and disadvantaged. We have seen how some life experiences that are excluding for wider populations affect people with dementia, sometimes in an exacerbated way, and how some experiences are unique to people with dementia. We have similarly seen how some aspects of services that are excluding for wider populations affect people with dementia, again sometimes in an exacerbated way, and how some service issues are very specifically related to dementia.

We have been reminded that we need to take into account the importance of age, class, sexuality, gender, ethnicity and race in understanding a continuum of experience from the multiply marginalised to the multiply privileged; that we need to understand 'interlocking oppressions'. Another side is that inclusion is not necessarily an 'all or nothing' – different people with dementia at different times may experience different degrees of inclusion and exclusion in different aspects of their lives.

The disability movement alerts us to the need to recognise commonality of interest in overcoming oppression as a basis for collective responses, and to the importance of not allowing concerns about segmentation and differentiation to detract from this. Referring to Campbell and Oliver (1996), Oliver and Barnes (1998, p.100) argue:

> ...the commonality among different groups is not otherness but the experience of oppression under capitalism. Collective resistance, and, indeed, collective reconstruction, must be organised around the different ways that experience manifests itself, and a genuine desire to end our own sectional oppressions by challenging all oppression. The disabled people's movement has made a formidable start in this direction by organising a collective movement within an oppressed population which is characterised by difference in terms of impairments and degrees of impairment, gender, class, ethnicity, sexuality and age, but who are united in their opposition to disability; the disabling tendencies of a modern society.

Alongside this, however, others have pointed to the importance of not glossing over differences between the experiences of different types of impairment, different conditions of onset and differences related to race, class and gender (Shakespeare 1993).

Overall the causes of, and experiences of, social exclusion affecting people with dementia are multifaceted and complex. It is well established that we cannot, and should not, think about people with dementia as a homogeneous group. Less well established is the extent to which people with dementia, or sub-populations of people with dementia, perceive themselves as having commonality of interest with each other or with other disadvantaged groups. A much greater understanding of how people with dementia perceive their interests will be important to inform policy and service responses and in understanding the potential for more collective action that we discuss below.

The goal of inclusion

It is important that we are clear conceptually about the nature of the inclusion advocated. Otherwise, it is easy to slip into ways of thinking and acting that are more about integration and conformity to social norms rather than promoting genuine recognition of diversity and equal rights. There are further lessons here that can be learnt from disability studies. Thus, Drake (1999) argues that the opposite of social exclusion is citizenship, which involves civil, political and social rights including having the opportunity to participate in core functions such as work, leisure, political debate and religious observance. Following from this, he argues that the goal of disability policies should be to extend disabled people's access to citizenship.

Drake (1999) points out that the pursuit of citizenship involves equality of opportunity and process, although not necessarily of outcome which may be affected by the individual's inherent limitations. Thus, one way in which we might assess our success in countering the social exclusion of people with dementia is to ask how far we enable people with dementia to maintain their citizenship.

This notion of citizenship, as Drake (1999, p.43) points out, is significantly different from notions of consumerism, where the 'exercise of power is limited to a particular set of predefined choices or even merely to the expression of a preference'. Citizenship therefore provides a more encompassing and challenging goal for the inclusion and empowerment of people with dementia than is entailed in many of the service development strategies which we will discuss later.

Current initiatives aim to enhance the citizenship and social participation of older people. The Better Government for Older People (BGOP) programme is an apparent success in achieving its aims of better meeting the needs of older people through a process of active engagement and consultation. BGOP moves away from the stereotyping of older people as 'service users' rather than full citizens (Thornton 2000). Godfrey and Callaghan (2000) also welcome approaches to consultation which focus on people's own views and experiences, emphasising the importance of participation in valued social activities, the maintenance of networks and continuity of place. The evaluation report on BGOP (Hayden and Boaz 2000) however acknowledges that people with dementia have yet to be included in initiatives such as these.

Service specialisation

One service strategy often advanced for achieving greater social inclusion is to target specific excluded groups or issues for special attention. This approach, in the form of recommendations for the development of specialist services for particular groups of people with dementia, has been raised at several points in the book.

Targeting particularly disadvantaged groups of people with dementia for special attention potentially has some obvious advantages in enabling care to be more finely tuned to their specific needs and circumstances. Specialisation can also make dementia care work more attractive if it brings additional resources and enhanced status for staff who develop advanced skills. However, there are also issues and potential problems that we need to take into account (see Percy-Smith 2000).

There are questions about who should decide on the groups and issues that should receive specialist attention and on what basis such decisions should be made. This is especially significant in the context of finite budgets when additional resources for a specific group may have knock-on effects on other services. There are potential difficulties in that groups defined on one count are not necessarily homogeneous on other important counts. There are likely to be overlaps between groups and people can fall into several groups at once. Membership of some target groups may be a passing phase in the lives of some people with dementia. There are risks of reinforcing negative or stereotyped perceptions and hence increasing the exclusion of targeted groups. There are risks that by targeting some groups we effectively 'miss out' or marginalise others. Finally, and very importantly for any strategy for inclusion, people may not see themselves as belonging to a 'group' even through others categorise them as fitting the objective criteria.

For example, in recent years younger people with dementia have been recognised as a marginalised group and targeted for attention. This has brought some very valuable benefits but also raised issues that illustrate many of the points above (see Tindall and Manthorpe 1997). The undoubted advantages of such targeting have included: much wider recognition that dementia does not just affect older people and that younger people have some needs that are different from older people; and the development of some services to more effectively meet the needs of younger people. However, dilemmas and debates remain about the arbitrariness of age boundaries, especially where these affect entitlement to services, and the need to recognise that younger people with dementia are not a homogeneous group.

This is not to argue against all specialisation and targeting. It is rather to suggest that we need to consider fully the intended and potential unintended consequences of such strategies. This includes the potential risk of creating more service boundaries and professional 'specialisms' that further fragment a service system in which co-ordination is a well-recognised problem (Audit Commission 2000, 2002). The challenge is similar to that described by Dunn (1999) in relation to mental health needs: '...the necessity of a constant "balancing act" between recognising difference while according equal treatment, countering fragmentation while supporting diversity' (Dunn 1999, p.64).

It includes the potential risk of marginalising the 'ordinary', the person with dementia who does not have particularly complex or challenging problems but whose life experience could nonetheless be improved. Similarly we need to consider the effect that 'special projects' may have, inadvertently or deliberately, of detracting attention from the many quality, staffing and resource problems of mainstream dementia services. For as Daker-White *et al.* (2002, p.113) point out, 'the key to improving services for marginalised groups lies in improving services for everybody with dementia and their carers'.

Policy development

Social policies designed specifically to promote social inclusion are largely about social cohesion and economic efficiency. These policies not surprisingly largely ignore groups, such as older people (including people with dementia), who are outside the labour market and pose no threat to social order or the moral consensus (Burden and Hamm 2000). These factors have contributed to the much greater political and resource commitment to implementation of the National Service Framework (NSF) for Mental Health (Department of Health 1999) than to the NSF for Older People (Department of Health 2001) which includes the standards for dementia services.

Given the multiple and interacting dimensions of the social exclusion of people with dementia we should not underestimate the scale and complexity of the policy task and the range of health, social care and other organisations that would have to be involved in working together to develop and implement a more inclusive policy framework (Graham *et al.* 2003).

People with dementia are seldom the subject of policy statements *per se* (Cantley 2001). It could be argued that in order to increase their social inclusion we should treat them as a distinct group for policy purposes. However, there are risks in this, as we noted in the discussion of specialisation in services.

The lives of people with dementia are affected by an enormous range of health and welfare policies as well as wider policies that shape the communities in which they live. People with dementia share many interests in common with other disadvantaged populations. If we are to achieve greater social inclusion for people with dementia then we must ensure that they are not excluded from the wider policy debates that concern them and that these wider policy debates encompass the diversity of experience within and between disadvantaged groups, including people with dementia.

Advocacy and collective action

The main 'user' organisations representing the interests of those affected by dementia in the UK are the Alzheimer's Society and Alzheimer Scotland – Action on Dementia. While these organisations have had substantial achievements in raising awareness of the needs of people with dementia and their families with the general public and policy makers, their impact on promoting the social inclusion of people with dementia has been much more limited. The membership of these organisations has traditionally mainly consisted of carers. It is therefore carers' perspectives and concerns that have been to the fore – perspectives and concerns that have to a considerable extent been underpinned by biomedical models, and often paternalistic assumptions, about the needs and potential of people with dementia. This is beginning to change with people with dementia increasingly being enabled to play an active role in the activities and management of the organisations.

Within research, and at the leading edges of practice development, there has been a good deal of attention paid to how, at an individual level, we can better 'hear the voice' of people with dementia expressing their views and feelings about the lives they want to live and the services they want to receive (Moriarty and Webb 2000; Wilkinson 2002). There has also been growing recognition that many people with dementia, often as a result of their impairment compounded by disempowerment, need the assistance of an advocate to ensure that their views and feelings are taken into account. Carers have often been regarded as the 'natural advocates' for people with dementia but it is increasingly being recognised that we should not assume that people with dementia and their carers share the same views and interests. We are therefore seeing growth in dementia advocacy services (Cantley, Steven and Smith 2003; Killeen 1996), a move that is supported by more general policy commitments to advocacy for service users. While this is to be welcomed, there are some important questions about different models of advocacy and the extent to which people with dementia can and should be included in the ownership of the developing schemes.

Also, in line with a more general UK policy thrust for 'user involvement' in services, we are beginning to see some developments in the direct involvement of people with dementia. There are a small but growing number of examples of services consulting with people with dementia and including individuals with dementia on planning and management groups (Innes et al. 2003). As yet there is no significant movement of people with dementia speaking out to influence public opinion, policy and services.

The emergence of Dementia Advocacy International, an Internet-based organisation of 'autonomous and competent people diagnosed with dementia, and our loyal allies' who are working together for improved quality of life, demonstrates that people with dementia can organise and act together. Such initiatives, although few and small scale, give rise to questions about the wider potential for collective action by people with dementia in countering social exclusion. Earlier and more accurate diagnosis means that more people with dementia are being identified at a stage when the nature of their impairment makes this much easier. In other fields such as physical disability, learning disability and mental health, the collective voices and actions of users/survivors play a very important role. However, such involvement is not universally welcomed by all service users (Small and Rhodes 2000) and we have yet to see the extent to which people with dementia will choose to take on roles as advocates or activists beyond their immediate personal interests.

Finally, thinking about the possibility of a movement of people with dementia brings us back to the theme of difference and commonality. Would there be risks of some dementia voices, most likely those of people with early dementia and younger people with dementia, dominating to the exclusion of those who are more disadvantaged? And would a movement of people with dementia see itself as having common cause with other excluded groups?

Conclusion

We have argued that if we are to achieve greater social inclusion of people with dementia we should increasingly think in terms of ensuring people's rights as citizens as well as their personhood; and in terms of community development and political activism as well as service development. We have also suggested that social inclusion requires 'joined up' action at different levels (individual, group, community, society) and the involvement of different stakeholders, including people with dementia, carers, service providers, managers, community leaders and politicians. Crucially, people with dementia themselves need to be actively engaged in 'owning' and shaping initiatives to promote their social inclusion at individual, community, service and policy levels.

Work in other fields suggests that promoting social inclusion for disadvantaged groups can bring benefits to us all through the community networks, participation, fairness, trust and reciprocity that is generated (e.g. Dunn 1999; Oliver and Barnes 1998). The challenge should not be underestimated:

> …a successful outcome might only be achieved by the further development of a bottom-up approach to policymaking, and a general acceptance that meaningful inclusion for disabled people, and, indeed, for other disadvantaged groups, is only possible through deep-rooted and radical changes in the way our society is organised. (Oliver and Barnes 1998, p.92)

References

Audit Commission (2000) *Forget Me Not: Mental Health Services for Older People.* London: Audit Commission.

Audit Commission (2002) *Forget Me Not 2002: Developing Mental Health Services for Older People in England.* London: Audit Commission.

Burden, T. and Hamm, T. (2000) 'Responding to socially excluded groups.' In J. Percy-Smith (ed) *Policy Responses to Social Exclusion: Towards Inclusion?* Buckingham: Open University Press.

Campbell, J. and Oliver, M. (1996) *Disability Politics: Understanding Our Past, Changing Our Future.* London and New York: Routledge.

Cantley, C. (2001) 'Understanding the policy context.' In C. Cantley (ed) *A Handbook of Dementia Care.* Buckingham: Open University Press.

Cantley, C., Steven, K. and Smith, M. (2003) *'Hear What I Say': Developing Dementia Advocacy Services.* Newcastle upon Tyne: Dementia North, Northumbria University.

Daker-White, G., Beattie, A., Means, R. and Gilliard, J. (2002) *Serving the Needs of Marginalised Groups in Dementia Care: Younger People and Minority Ethnic Groups.* Bristol: University of the West of England and Dementia Voice.

Dementia Advocacy International (no date) www.dasninternational.org

Department of Health (1999) *National Service Framework for Mental Health Modern Standards and Service Models.* London: Department of Health.

Department of Health (2001) *National Service Framework for Older People.* London: Department of Health.

Drake, R.F. (1999) *Understanding Disability Policies.* Basingstoke and London: Macmillan Press.

Dunn, S. (1999) *Creating Accepting Communities: Report of the Mind Inquiry into Social Exclusion and Mental Health Problems.* London: Mind Publications.

Godfrey, M. and Callaghan, G. (2000) *Exploring Unmet Need: The Challenge of a User-Centred Response.* York: Joseph Rowntree Foundation.

Graham, N., Lindesay, J., Katona, C., Bertolote, J.M., Camus, V., Copeland, J.R.M., de Mendonça Lima, C.A., Gaillard, M., Gély Nargeot, M.C., Gray, J., Jacobsson, L. Kingma, M., Kühne, N., O'Loughlin, A., Rutz, W., Saraceno, B., Taintor, Z. and Wancata, J. (2003) 'Reducing stigma and discrimination against older people with mental disorders: a technical consensus statement.' *International Journal of Geriatric Psychiatry 18,* 670–678.

Hayden, C. and Boaz, A. (2000) *Making a Difference: Better Government for Older People Evaluation Report.* www.bgop.org.uk/pages/evaluation_reports.html

Innes, A., Stalker, K., Ferguson, I., Brownlie, J., Archibald, C., Hubbard, G., Simmons, R., Jones, C., Petrie, M., Ribeiro, P., Anderson, I. and MacDonald, C. (2003) *Seeking Users' Views in Service Delivery and Organisation Research.* Unpublished report to the National Co-ordinating Centre for NHS Service Delivery and Organisation R&D (NCC SDO).

Killeen, J. (1996) *Advocacy and Dementia.* Edinburgh: Alzheimer Scotland – Action on Dementia.

Moriarty, J. and Webb, S. (2000) *Part of their Lives: Community Care for Older People with Dementia.* Bristol: Policy Press.

Oliver, M. and Barnes, C. (1998) *Disabled People and Social Policy: From Exclusion to Inclusion.* Longman Social Policy in Britain Series. Harlow, Essex: Addison Wesley Longman.

Percy-Smith, J. (2000) 'Introduction: the contours of social exclusion.' In J. Percy-Smith (ed) *Policy Responses to Social Exclusion: Towards Inclusion?* Buckingham: Open University Press.

Sapey, B. (2001) 'From stigma to the social exclusion of disabled people.' In T. Mason, C. Carlisle, C. Watkins and E. Whitehead (eds) *Stigma and Social Exclusion in Healthcare.* London and New York: Routledge.

Shakespeare, T. (1993) 'Disabled people's self-organisation: a new social movement?' *Disability, Handicap and Society 8,* 3, 249–264.

Small, N. and Rhodes, P. (2000) *Too Ill to Talk? User Involvement in Palliative Care.* London and New York: Routledge.

Thornton, P. (2000) *Older People Speaking Out: Developing Opportunities for Influence.* York: Joseph Rowntree Foundation.

Tindall, L. and Manthorpe, J. (1997) 'Early onset dementia: a case of ill-timing?' *Journal of Mental Health 6,* 3, 237–249.

Wilkinson, H. (ed) (2002) *The Perspectives of People with Dementia: Research Methods and Motivations.* London: Jessica Kingsley Publishers.

The Contributors

Carole Archibald is a registered nurse and health visitor who in 2002 was awarded a PhD on the subject of sexuality and dementia. She has worked in the field of dementia for the past 18 years, initially as a specialist health visitor, then for the past 14 years as a Senior Fieldworker at the Dementia Services Development Centre at the University of Stirling. She has provided consultancy and training and undertaken research on dementia issues during this time and has published widely on topics that include sexuality, activities, specialist dementia units, respite and people with dementia in acute hospitals.

Clive Ballard has recently taken up a post as Professor of Age Related Disorders at the Institute of Psychiatry, King's College London, having previously been Professor of Old Age Psychiatry at the University of Newcastle. Ongoing programmes of research include vascular dementia, dementia with Lewy bodies, psychiatric and behavioural symptoms in people with dementia and the use of sedative drugs in people with dementia. He has published widely in these areas.

Professor Colin Bell (1942–2003) was a distinguished sociologist with particular scholarly interests in social mobility, family and marriage, stratification and power, and research methodology. He also made a significant academic contribution to a wide range of policy issues including agriculture, environment, employment relationships, race and ethnic relations, and access to higher education. He took up office as Principal and Vice-Chancellor of the University of Stirling in September 2001. He was previously Vice-Chancellor and Principal of the University of Bradford. From 1988 Colin Bell was Professor of Sociology at the University of Edinburgh, where he also served as Vice-Principal from 1993 to 1998.

John Bond is Professor of Social Gerontology and Health Services Research at the University of Newcastle and specialises on researching the psychosocial and economic aspects of dementia and contributing to clinical trials of interventions for older people. He is Director of the Centre for Health Services Research and a member of the Institute for Ageing and Health.

Alison Bowes is Professor of Sociology and Head of the Department of Applied Social Science at the University of Stirling. Her main research interests concern minority ethnic groups and older people's experiences of and views about health, housing and social care services, with particular reference to their implications for social justice.

Michael Bradbury has worked for the Institute for Ageing and Health based at Newcastle General Hospital for the past two years. He has been working as an assistant psychologist, under the supervision of Professor Clive Ballard and Professor Rose Anne Kenny, on the 'Memory after Stroke Study'. He studied psychology at the University of Wales, Swansea, and completed a Masters degree in research methods in psychology at the University of Bristol.

Errollyn Bruce joined Bradford Dementia Group to work with family carers, which led to interests in reminiscence work and attachment dynamics in caring relationships. Her chapter is based on data from a study of well-being among people with dementia living in long-term care. She is now a lecturer in Dementia Studies at the University of Bradford.

Caroline Cantley is Professor of Dementia Care at Northumbria University and Director of Dementia North, a regional dementia services development centre. Her professional background is in social work and she has experience as a manager in social services and in health services. Her work as a university teacher and researcher has been in the fields of mental health, services for older people and, most recently, dementia care.

Rik Cheston is a consultant clinical psychologist working with older people in west Wiltshire, as part of the Avon and Wiltshire Mental Health Partnership. He is the co-author, with Michael Bender, of *Understanding Dementia: The Man with the Worried Eyes*, also published by Jessica Kingsley Publishers.

Noni Cobban was the project leader for the Raising the Standard Project at the Dementia Services Development Centre, University of Stirling. She is a qualified nurse with a diploma in community care studies. She has many years' experience in the provision of care at home services for older people and people with dementia mainly in the independent sector. Her current interest is the support, supervision and development of frontline home care staff.

Lynne Corner is an Alzheimer's Society Research Fellow and is based at the Centre for Health Services Research and Institute for Ageing and Health, University of Newcastle upon Tyne. Dr Corner has a background in health services research for older people and a particular interest in the health and social care of older people with dementia and their carers and quality of life assessment.

Sylvia Cox is Planning Consultant with the Dementia Centre at the University of Stirling and previously worked for 25 years as a social work senior manager in child care, adult and elderly people's services. Her current responsibilities include development, consultancy and evaluation on user involvement, assessment and care management, housing and support, complex needs and end of life care. She has published on younger people with dementia, end of life care and dementia in rural and remote areas. Sylvia is a member of the Joseph Rowntree Foundation Task Group on 'Housing, Care and Money' for older people, chair of the Expert Group on Alcohol Related Brain Damage and a director of Carr-Gomm Scotland.

Claire Craig is a qualified occupational therapist and has spent a number of years working with people with dementia. During this time she has been particularly interested in the role of the arts as a vehicle for communication and in the way that the environment can support the individual. Claire has written about these ideas in the publications *Creative Environments* and *Celebrating the Person*, both of which have been published by the Dementia Services Development Centre, Stirling. Claire has recently been appointed as a Senior Lecturer in Occupational Therapy at Sheffield Hallam University, where she hopes to be able to develop and share these ideas further.

Peggye Dilworth-Anderson is Director of the Center for Ageing and Diversity, UNC Institute on Ageing and Professor of Health Policy and Administration in the School of Public Health at the University of North Carolina at Chapel Hill. She has received numerous awards and recognitions for her work during her career. She is a fellow of the Gerontological Society of America, National Council on Family Relations and the Cecil G. Sheps Research Center on Health Services Research at the University of North Carolina at Chapel Hill. She currently serves on three editorial boards: *Journal of Gerontology: Social Sciences, Journal of Aging and Mental Health* and *Psychology and Aging.*

Andrew Fairbairn arrived in Newcastle as a medical student in 1968 and has had at least one foot there ever since! He is an Old Age Psychiatrist, has been a Senior Policy Adviser to the Department of Health, is a member of the NHS Taskforce for Older People and chaired the Mental Health Foundation's Mental Illness in Later Life Advisory Group. He is currently Medical Director of Newcastle, North Tyneside and Northumberland Mental Health NHS Trust and Registrar of the Royal College of Psychiatrists.

Ruth Graham is a Research Associate and Public Health Tutor at the University of Newcastle (School of Surgical and Reproductive Medicine, and School of Population and Health Sciences). Her work on cognitive citizenship forms part of a broader research focus on social justice and healthcare.

Wendy Hulko is a PhD Candidate and Teaching Assistant in the Department of Applied Social Science at the University of Stirling in Scotland. Prior to doctoral studies, Wendy worked for several years with older people and people with dementia in clinical (social work and nursing), research and policy settings in Canada. She obtained her Masters of Social Work degree in 1998. These experiences contributed to her interest in the socio-cultural context of dementia, subjective experiences of dementia, and intersectionality/interlocking oppressions.

Anthea Innes is Senior Lecturer in Dementia Studies in the Department of Applied Social Science at the University of Stirling. Prior to this, she was a lecturer with Bradford Dementia Group. Her primary research interest is dementia and dementia care. She is particularly interested in groups that are marginalised, including minority ethnic groups, unqualified care staff and people with dementia in rural areas.

John Killick, a former teacher, was from 1992 to 2003 Writer in Residence for Westminster Health Care. From 1998 he has also been Research Fellow in Communication Through the Arts in the Dementia Services Development Centre at the University of Stirling. His collections of 'Dementia Poems' have been published by Hawker, and he is co-author with Kate Allan of *Communication and the Care of People with Dementia*.

Jill Manthorpe is Professor of Social Work at King's College London and Co-Director of the Social Care Workforce Research Unit. She has undertaken a variety of research projects on risk and has written a distance learning text on the subject for the Open University (with Nicky Stanley), as well as articles and books for professional readerships in health and social care (with Andy Alaszewski). Other current research includes the area of intermediate care, older workers, food and dementia, disabled students and adult protection. Recent books are *Dementia Care*, edited with Trevor Adams, and *The Age of the Inquiry*, edited with Nicky Stanley. Jill is co-editor of *Practice* and of *Research, Policy and Planning*, and vice-chair of the Social Services Research Group.

Gillian McColgan is a Sociologist and Research Fellow at the University of Stirling. Her PhD work was an ethnography in a private nursing home where research informants were people who had dementia. Her continuing interests are in ethics in research, relationships and social support, with a particular interest in companion animals as social support and assistance animals in everyday life.

Christian Müller-Hergl is a registered nurse and has written numerous articles about DCM and nursing philosophy. He currently works as a teacher and trainer at the Meinwerk-Institut in Paderborn, where he trains nurses in gerontopsychiatry and psychogerontology, and supervises teams working in Special Care Units (SCUs) for people with dementia and depression.

Charlie Murphy has worked for the Dementia Services Development Centre at the University of Stirling for the past 11 years. His interests include the voice of people with dementia; life-story work; and evaluations of community services for people with dementia. He contributed to *The Person with Alzheimer's Disease: Pathways to Understanding the Experience*, edited by P.B. Harris.

Kirsty Sherlock is currently employed at the Macaulay Institute as part of the Socio-Economics Research Programme where she researches participatory processes for land use and environmental management. This allows her to continue her research interests in gender, rural sustainability, policy processes, environmental justice and giving voice. For further information, please contact her on k.sherlock@macaulay.ac.uk.

Karen Watchman is Director of Down's Syndrome Scotland and an Associate Lecturer with the Open University School of Health and Social Welfare. Her research interests include Down's Syndrome and dementia and end of life issues for people with a learning disability. She has an interest in working alongside people with Down's Syndrome to further their inclusion in the research process.

Subject Index

Author Index